NATURAL
REMEDIES
SUSTAIN ME

Over 100 Herbal Remedies For Different Kinds of Ailments- What The BIG Pharma Doesn't Want You To Know!

Inspired By

Barbara O'Neill's

Teachings

Niella Brown

Disclaimer:

The information provided in this book is for informational purposes only. Please consult with your health care provider for medical advice. The author specifically disclaims any liability that is incurred from the use or application of the contents of this book

Table of Contents

INTRODUCTION

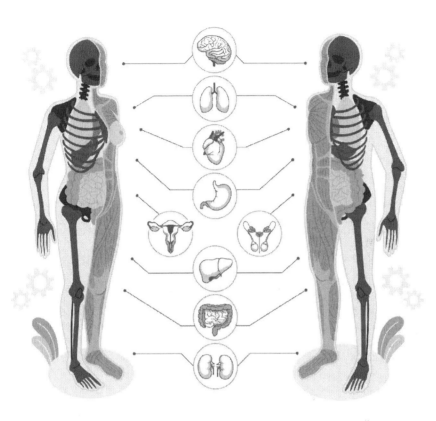

Today, our world is filled with countless remedies and treatments for various ailments imaginable and unimaginable, but in the midst of this, there emerges a voice that challenges the conventional wisdom. Barbara O'Neill, a trailblazing advocate for holistic health, has long been a beacon of controversy in the realm of wellness. Her radical belief? There are no external cures; there is only one cure—the human body itself.

My book: "Natural Remedies Sustain Me" was birthed from the belief that the body has the innate ability to heal itself.. This book is largely inspired by Barbara's unwavering conviction that God designed our bodies with an incredible capacity for self-restoration, provided we grant it the right conditions. But here's the catch—most of us remain blissfully ignorant of what those conditions truly entail.

In this handbook of natural remedies, l delved deep into the fundamental laws of health, addressing ailments from the crown of our heads to the tips of our toes. Prepare to be taken on an eye-opening journey, exploring how the body can rejuvenate itself. All you need to do is to open your mind to comprehend these fundamental principles.

While it might be challenging to pinpoint a singular solution for all, nevertheless as Barbara advised; each one of us can become our own doctor. We also need to take the following seriously such as hydration, restorative sleep, exercise, and nourishment from natural foods, but the magic lies more in the subtle adjustments unique to each individual. Importantly, Listen to your body, make adjustments and then listen again.

The lost art of listening to our bodies takes center stage in this captivating exploration of self-healing. In a world overwhelmed with external fixes, "Natural Remedies Sustain Me" reminds us that the most potent cure resides within.

Prepare to embark on a journey of self-discovery, empowerment, and holistic well-being, where the body becomes the ultimate guide, whispering its preferences, and leading you to a life of vibrant health.

Are you ready to rediscover the natural remedies of over a hundred ailments such as cancer, diabetes, leprosy, arthritis, obesity, fever, headache, insomnia, appendicitis, tumor, hepatitis, liver issues, kidney stones, malaria, tonsillitis, pile, hernia, asthma, pneumonia, tuberculosis, gonorrhea, urinary challenges, syphilis, goiter, acne, ulcer, endometriosis, erectile dysfunction, mumps, measles, smallpox, typhoid fever, burns & Injuries, common cold, body pain etc.

Then stay with me on this ride as we embark on a transformative quest to unlock the healing potential within.

100 NATURAL REMEDIES
(What BIG Pharma Doesn't Want You to Know)

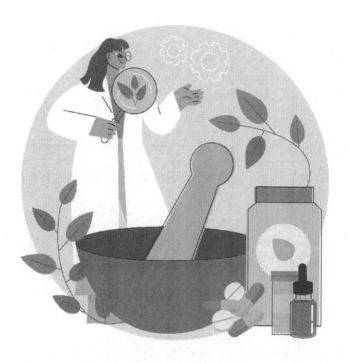

Hypertension (High Blood Pressure)

Hypertension, commonly known as high blood pressure, increases gradually with age, often changing in patterns between genders over the years. While there's a natural range of blood pressure, a young adult's average is around 120/80 mm Hg. Several factors contribute to hypertension: overeating leading to obesity, a diet high in salt, and strain on the liver and kidneys due to excessive irritating foods. In many cases, hypertension can be hereditary. Symptoms like morning headaches, difficulty breathing, dizziness, a flushed complexion, and blurred vision are common. It's a significant risk factor for heart failure, strokes, and heart attacks.

Root Causes

The primary contributors to hypertension include poor dietary choices, particularly those high in salt and stimulants, and lifestyle factors like obesity and tobacco use. Stress, lack of rest, and excessive physical and social activities also play a significant role, leading to increased blood pressure.

Natural remedy

To manage hypertension, herbal remedies can be effective. Herbs like golden seal, red clover, wild cherry bark, vervain, and others have been identified as beneficial. Golden seal, for instance, can be consumed by adding a teaspoon to boiling water and drinking it several times a day. Red clover tea is recommended for blood purification. These herbs work to cleanse the body and support cardiovascular health.

Herbal Potion

To prepare an effective herbal remedy for hypertension:

- **Golden Seal Potion**: Add one teaspoon of golden seal to a pint of boiling water. Consume a small amount at least six times a day.
- **Red Clover Tea**: Replace regular water intake with red clover tea. Brew the tea by steeping red clover flowers in hot water.

Additionally, maintaining a diet free from white flour, cane sugar, meats, and stimulants like caffeine, and incorporating fruits, outdoor exercise, deep breathing, and adequate rest are crucial. Warm baths and herbal teas that induce sleep can also help in lowering blood pressure. Regular exercise, managing salt intake, and maintaining a healthy weight are essential preventative measures. If blood pressure remains high, seeking medical advice is recommended.

Low blood pressure (Hypotension)

Low blood pressure, or hypotension, is a condition often overlooked yet significant. Modern understanding categorizes it as blood pressure lower than 110/70 mmHg. It's prevalent in adults who may have a consistent systolic pressure ranging between 90 to 100 mmHg. Recognizing this condition is crucial as it reflects the body's need for better nourishment and overall vitality.

Root cause

The root cause of hypotension can be attributed to inadequate nutrition, lack of rest, insufficient exercise, and conditions leading to reduced vitality, such as blood loss or certain neurological and muscular diseases. Addressing these underlying issues is key to managing low blood pressure.

Natural remedy

These include herbs like **hyssop, golden seal, vervain, prickly ash, blue cohosh, gentian, wood betony, burnet,** and **skullcap**. Adding a small amount of red pepper to these herbs can enhance their vitality-boosting properties.

To prepare a herbal potion for low blood pressure, one can create a blend using any of these herbs. Here's a simple method:

1. Choose one or more herbs from the list: hyssop, golden seal, vervain, prickly ash, blue cohosh, gentian, wood betony, burnet, or skullcap.

2. Mix a teaspoon of the chosen herb(s) with a pinch of red pepper.

3. Steep this mixture in hot water for about 10 minutes to make an herbal tea.

4. Strain and consume this tea daily.

Diet plays a pivotal role in managing low blood pressure. A diet rich in nourishing foods like potassium broth, mashed potatoes, baked potatoes (with skin), soybean milk, soy cottage cheese, leafy vegetables, and a variety of other vegetables is recommended. Avoiding de-vitaminized or stimulating foods and opting for digestion-friendly options like peppermint or spearmint tea can also be beneficial. Drinking liquids during meals should be minimized to prevent digestion issues.

Regular outdoor exercise is essential for normalizing blood pressure. Additionally, Echinacea, known for its blood-toning properties, can be taken in capsule form (one capsule, three times a day) as a supplementary measure.

Acute Myocardial Infarction (Heart Attack)

Acute myocardial infarction, commonly known as a heart attack, occurs when blood flow to a part of the heart is blocked for a long enough period that part of the heart muscle is damaged or dies. This is usually due to a buildup of plaque, a substance mostly made of fat, cholesterol, and cellular waste products, in the coronary arteries. This buildup narrows the arteries, reducing blood flow to the heart, and can ultimately lead to a heart attack.

Root Cause

The primary causes of a heart attack include coronary artery disease (the buildup of plaque in the arteries), smoking, high blood pressure, high cholesterol levels, obesity, a sedentary lifestyle, and diabetes. Poor diet, stress, and excessive alcohol consumption also contribute. Genetics and age can also be factors, with risk increasing as one gets older.

Natural remedy

While immediate medical attention is crucial in the case of a heart attack, certain herbs and natural supplements can support heart health and potentially reduce the risk of heart issues. Herbs like **hawthorn, garlic,** and **turmeric** are known for their cardiovascular benefits. Hawthorn, for instance, is renowned for improving blood flow, reducing blood pressure, and enhancing heart functioning.

Preparation of Herbal Potion

1. **Hawthorn Tincture**: To prepare a hawthorn tincture, steep hawthorn berries, leaves, and flowers in a mixture of alcohol and water. This tincture can be taken in small doses daily.

2. **Garlic Infusion**: Add crushed garlic cloves to a jar and cover with an alcohol solution. Let it sit for several weeks, shaking it occasionally. Strain and take a small amount daily.

3. **Turmeric Tea**: Boil a teaspoon of turmeric powder in water for 10 minutes. Strain and drink this tea once daily.

Hemorrhages

Hemorrhages can manifest in different forms, such as bleeding from the lungs, uterus, bowels, and nose. Traditional remedies suggest the use of specific herbs for each type. For lung hemorrhages, herbs effective for stomach bleeding are recommended. Uterine bleeding can be managed by resting, elevating the legs, and using a douche prepared from bayberry bark or bistort root. Herbal teas from red raspberry leaves, white oak bark, witch hazel, or wild alum root are also beneficial. Bowel hemorrhages can be addressed with enemas using wild alum root, white oak bark, or red raspberry tea. Nosebleeds may be managed with a **golden seal tea or a combination of wild alum root, blackberry leaves, witch hazel leaves,** and **white oak bark**. While these remedies are often effective, persistent bleeding should be evaluated by a physician as it may indicate serious conditions like cancer.

Root Cause

The root cause of hemorrhages varies depending on the location but generally involves the rupture or weakness of blood vessels. Herbal treatments focus on astringent properties to constrict blood vessels and reduce bleeding.

Natural remedy

Herbs like;

- Bayberry Bark
- Bistort Root
- Red Raspberry Leaves
- White Oak Bark
- Witch Hazel Bark
- Wild Alum Root
- Shepherd's Purse
- Sumac

- Golden Seal
- Blackberry Leaves

All these herbs have been known to help in managing hemorrhages. These herbs are celebrated for their astringent and healing properties, which aid in reducing bleeding and promoting recovery.

Herbal Potion

1. **For Lung and Uterine Hemorrhages:**
   - Steep 1 tablespoon of bayberry bark or bistort root in a quart of boiling water for a few minutes. For teas, use 2 tablespoons in a quart of boiling water, steep for 20 minutes, strain, and drink as hot as possible.

2. **For Bowel Hemorrhages:**
   - Prepare a tea with wild alum root, white oak bark, or red raspberry leaves. Inject 2-3 ounces of this tea as an enema, retaining it as long as possible.

3. **For Nosebleeds:**
   - Steep 1 teaspoon of golden seal in a pint of boiling water. Once cooled, use the tea to sniff up the nostrils. Alternatively, prepare a combination tea using wild alum root, blackberry leaves, witch hazel leaves, and white oak bark.

Deep Vein Thrombosis

Deep Vein Thrombosis (DVT) might sound like a condition straight out of a medical drama, but it's a real and often under-discussed health issue. Imagine this: blood clots forming deep within your veins, often in the legs. It's like a traffic jam in your bloodstream, where the flow is disrupted, causing swelling, pain, and a host of complications.

Root Cause

At its core, DVT is like a mystery with various suspects contributing to its occurrence. It's often linked to prolonged periods of inactivity – think long flights or bed rest – which slow down blood circulation. Add to that factors like certain medications, smoking, or conditions like obesity and heart disease, and you've got the perfect storm for DVT.

Natural remedy

Now, let's talk about the herbal guardians. These aren't your usual suspects; they're lesser-known but equally potent. Picture **Ginkgo Biloba**, a tree with ancient roots, its leaves improving blood circulation and reducing clot formation. **Hawthorn berries**, another ally, are like the cheerleaders of cardiovascular health, known to strengthen blood vessels. Then there's the **Horse Chestnut**, not your regular nut, but a seed that reduces swelling and improves blood flow.

Herbal Potion

Creating these potions requires a dash of patience and a sprinkle of care. Let's brew:

1. **Ginkgo Biloba Tea**: Steep dried ginkgo leaves in hot water for about 10 minutes. Strain and enjoy this mind-clarifying brew once daily. It's like a cup of historical wisdom, enhancing your blood flow.

2. **Hawthorn Berry Tonic**: Simmer dried hawthorn berries in water for 20 minutes. Strain and sip this heart-happy tonic twice a day. It's a drink that cheers to your blood vessels' health.

3. **Horse Chestnut Salve**: Grind the horse chestnut seeds into a powder and mix with a carrier oil. Apply this earthy paste to the affected area to reduce swelling and encourage circulation.

Varicose Veins

Varicose veins, often resulting from prolonged standing, sluggish circulation, pregnancy, or inherited factors, involve enlarged, knotted veins in the legs, causing pain and sometimes leading to skin ulcers. A nourishing diet, regular bowel movements, and cold baths can help manage this condition. Special stockings and topical applications like white oak bark tea can offer relief. For severe cases, a blend of **golden seal, myrrh, and a mix of hyssop, white cherry bark,** and **yellow dock root** can be taken. Herbs such as white oak bark, witch hazel, bayberry bark, wild alum root, and burnet are recommended.

Root Cause

The primary causes of varicose veins include factors like prolonged standing, poor circulation, pregnancy, and genetics. These factors lead to the enlargement and twisting of veins, causing discomfort and potential complications.

Natural remedy

The recommended herbal remedies include:

1. White Oak Bark

2. Witch Hazel

3. Bayberry Bark

4. Wild Alum Root

5. Burnet

Herbal Potion

1. **Golden Seal and Myrrh Tea**: Steep a heaping teaspoon of golden seal and a half teaspoon of myrrh in a pint of boiling water for 20 minutes. Consume six to seven times a day.

2. **Hyssop, White Cherry Bark, and Yellow Dock Root Mix**: Combine equal parts of powdered hyssop, white cherry bark, and yellow dock root. Take half a teaspoon in a quarter glass of cold water, followed by a glass of hot water, four times daily, an hour before meals and before bedtime.

3. **Topical Application**: For external application, particularly if there are ulcers, prepare a strong tea of white oak bark and apply it to the affected limbs two to three times before sleeping.

Pulmonary Embolism

Pulmonary embolism (PE) is a condition as old as time, yet it remains a critical concern in modern medicine. It occurs when a blood clot, often formed in the veins of the legs or pelvis, travels through the bloodstream and becomes lodged in the lungs. This blockage can be life-threatening, disrupting blood flow and affecting lung function.

Root Cause

The primary cause of PE is deep vein thrombosis (DVT) - blood clots forming in the deeper veins. Factors contributing to DVT include prolonged immobility (like long flights or bed rest), certain medical conditions, smoking, obesity, and genetic predispositions. These clots can break free and travel to the lungs, causing a pulmonary embolism.

Natural remedy

For herbal medicine, several herbs are believed to offer relief and healing properties for conditions like PE. The key players are **Pleurisy Root, Lobelia, Beth Root, Colombo,** and **Horehound.** These herbs have been used traditionally to improve respiratory health, reduce inflammation, and aid in blood circulation.

Herbal Potion

To create an herbal blend for potentially aiding in the management of pulmonary embolism, follow these steps:

1. **Pleurisy Root Tea**: Steep 1-2 teaspoons of dried Pleurisy Root in boiling water for 10 minutes. This herb is known for its ability to alleviate inflammation and aid in breathing.

2. **Lobelia Tincture**: This powerful herb can be used sparingly. Mix a few drops of Lobelia tincture with

water and take it once daily. Lobelia is known for its relaxing effect on the respiratory system.

3. **Beth Root Brew**: Simmer one teaspoon of dried Beth Root in a cup of water for about 15 minutes. Beth Root is traditionally used for its blood-stabilizing properties.

4. **Colombo Infusion**: Steep one teaspoon of dried Colombo root in hot water for 10 minutes. Colombo is known for aiding digestion and boosting overall health.

5. **Horehound Syrup**: Boil horehound leaves with water and honey to create a soothing syrup. Horehound has a long history of use for respiratory ailments.

Nosebleed

Nosebleeds, a common yet often alarming occurrence, can arise from various causes such as nasal injury, exposure to high heat or altitude, head congestion, or blood abnormalities. While traditional medical approaches are effective, it's important to recognize the power of herbal remedies, which have been successfully used for generations and are often overlooked by the pharmaceutical industry.

Root cause

The root cause of a nosebleed typically lies in the acute stress experienced by the nasal blood vessels. This can be due to physical trauma, environmental factors, or internal physiological changes. To address this, nature offers a bounty of herbs known for their healing properties.

Natural remedy

For a Natural remedy, consider these potent herbs: **golden seal, wild alum root, white oak bark, bayberry bark,** and **ephedra vulgaris**. These herbs have been known to provide relief not only for nosebleeds but also for sinus issues and colds, attesting to their versatility and effectiveness.

Herbal potion

1. **Golden Seal Solution**: Take a heaping teaspoon of golden seal and steep it in a pint of boiling soft or distilled water. Add boric acid to saturation (until no more dissolves). Let the mixture settle, then cool it. Sniff this solution several times a day until the bleeding stops.

2. **Wild Alum Root, White Oak Bark, or Bayberry Bark**: Use one heaping teaspoon of any of these herbs

per cup of boiling water. Steep for 30 minutes, then strain or let the sediment settle. Sniff the solution and use it as a gargle. Swallowing a small amount is harmless.

3. **Ephedra Vulgaris**: Steep one heaping teaspoon in a cup of boiling water for 30 minutes. Strain or let the sediment settle and then use it as a nasal sniff.

Using soft or distilled water is recommended for these preparations to ensure purity and effectiveness.

Migraines, cluster headaches

Migraines are debilitating headaches that drastically reduce the quality of life for those who suffer from them. They can be so overwhelming that sufferers often find themselves unable to tackle even the most basic tasks. While there are various types of headaches, the root causes often overlap.

Root Cause

One of the primary causes of migraines is thought to be infections and infestations in the body, such as tooth infections, urinary tract infections, bowel issues, and particularly the presence of a wormlet called Strongyloides. Additionally, certain food allergies, including reactions to dairy, eggs, citrus, and salty foods, can exacerbate migraine symptoms. However, avoiding these foods long-term is challenging.

Natural remedy

A more sustainable approach involves targeting the root causes directly. This can be done using herbs and natural remedies. For example, to address the issue of Strongyloides, a parasite cleanse using herbal remedies can be effective. For dental infections, rinsing with a solution made from white iodine or Lugol can help. Regular bowel cleansing, possibly using herbs like **Cascara sagrada or senna tea**, is recommended for maintaining digestive health. Additionally, liver cleanses using natural methods can help detoxify the body and reduce migraine triggers.

How to Make the Herbal Potion:

1. **For Strongyloides and Bacteria:** A simple herbal parasite cleanse can be made by combining **wormwood, black walnut hull,** and **cloves**. These herbs are known to be effective against various parasites and can be consumed in tincture or tea form.

2. **For Dental Infections:** Mix 12 drops of white iodine or 6 drops of Lugol's in ¼ cup of water. Use this solution to rinse the mouth, especially around any affected teeth.

3. **For Bowel Cleansing:** Brew a tea using Cascara sagrada or senna leaves. Steep the leaves in hot water for about 10 minutes and consume before bedtime.

4. **Liver Cleanse:** A simple liver cleanse involves drinking a mixture of olive oil, lemon juice, and garlic. This should be done periodically to maintain liver health.

In conclusion, while migraines can be caused by various factors, addressing underlying infections and imbalances with herbal remedies can offer substantial relief.

Infant Paralysis (Poliomyelitis)

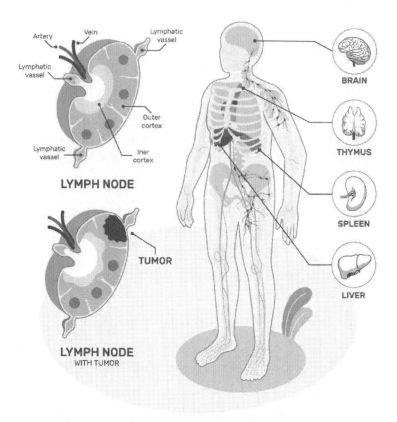

Infantile paralysis, or poliomyelitis, is a viral disease spread through human contact, entering the body via the mouth and affecting the intestines, lymph nodes, and nervous system. Its early symptoms are often non-specific, including fever, fatigue, muscle aches, and sometimes gastrointestinal issues. More severe symptoms like muscle weakness and paralysis can follow. While vaccination has nearly eradicated polio in many regions, traditional herbal remedies have also shown promising results in managing its symptoms.

Root Cause

The root cause of poliomyelitis is a virus that enters the body through the mouth, predominantly affecting the intestines before potentially impacting the lymphatic system and nervous system.

Natural remedy

Herbal remedies have been used successfully to support the treatment of poliomyelitis symptoms. These include:

- Prickly Ash Berries
- Wild Cherry Bark
- English/American Valerian Root
- Poplar Bark
- Dandelion Root
- Skullcap
- Golden Seal
- Black Cohosh
- Catnip
- Red Clover
- Yellow Dock

These herbs have been hidden gems, with many cured by their use, a fact often overshadowed by the pharmaceutical industry's focus on more commercial treatments.

Herbal Potion

An effective herbal tea can be made by mixing equal parts of the selected herbs. For instance, a blend of valerian, catnip, and calamus root can be prepared as follows:

1. Mix one tablespoon each of valerian, catnip, and calamus root.

2. Steep one teaspoon of this mixture in a cup of boiling water.

3. Consume one-fourth of a cup every two hours. The tea is safe in larger quantities.

4. For children, administer the tea in tablespoon doses several times a day, sweetened with honey or malt sugar.

Additionally, an antispasmodic tincture, administered in doses of 8-15 drops in a quarter glass of hot water, can be beneficial, with dosage adjusted for age.

Sleep Apnea

Sleep apnea, a condition characterized by interrupted breathing during sleep, is often linked to environmental and internal factors. Key contributors include air toxins like cigarette smoke, vanadium from gas leaks, chemicals from new carpets or treated fabrics, and possibly asbestos or formaldehyde. These toxins can lead to swollen throat tissues, narrowing the air passage and causing difficulty in breathing. Apart from environmental toxins, allergic reactions, including food and drug allergies or a lack of vitamin C, can also cause throat swelling. Additionally, infections from bacteria or viruses may contribute to the condition. Persistent metals in the mouth can affect throat immunity, exacerbating the problem. While obesity is commonly cited as a cause, it's not universally applicable, especially in infants. Addressing these potential causes is crucial for managing sleep apnea.

Root Cause

The primary root causes of sleep apnea are environmental toxins, allergies, and infections, leading to throat swelling and restricted airways.

Natural remedy

A holistic approach involves using herbs that can help reduce throat swelling and boost immunity. Herbs such as **turmeric** (for its anti-inflammatory properties), **echinacea** (to boost immunity), and **licorice root** (for soothing the throat) are beneficial.

How to Make the Herbal Potion:

- **Turmeric Tea:**
    1. Boil 1 cup of water and add 1 teaspoon of ground turmeric.

2. Simmer for 10 minutes and strain.

3. Add honey to taste and drink warm.

- **Echinacea Tincture:**

    1. Mix 1 part echinacea root with 5 parts alcohol (like vodka).

    2. Seal in a jar and store in a cool, dark place for about 4 weeks, shaking daily.

    3. After 4 weeks, strain and store in a dropper bottle. Use as directed.

- **Licorice Root Tea:**

    1. Boil 1 cup of water and add 1 teaspoon of dried licorice root.

    2. Steep for 5-10 minutes, strain, and drink.

Alzheimer's disease and Dementia

Alzheimer's disease and Dementia are often associated with aging, but they're not necessarily caused by it. Mental deterioration in the elderly is largely attributed to a decline in the liver's ability to detoxify toxins. These toxins, more impactful in the elderly, can lead to symptoms like memory loss, disorientation, and physical instability. The key to combating these symptoms lies in reducing exposure to common toxins, particularly in diet, environment, and overall lifestyle. For the elderly, especially those showing signs of mental deterioration, significant lifestyle changes can lead to noticeable improvements in their health and quality of life.

Root Cause

The root cause of the symptoms commonly associated with aging, such as memory loss and disorientation, is the decreased efficiency of the liver in detoxifying harmful substances. As we age, our liver's capability to process toxins diminishes, resulting in these toxins circulating in the body and affecting brain function and overall health.

Natural remedy

Herbs like **milk thistle, dandelion root,** and **turmeric** are renowned for their ability to support liver function and aid in detoxification. Incorporating these herbs into one's diet can help in mitigating the effects of toxins on the body and brain.

Preparation of Herbal Potion

To prepare a detoxifying herbal potion:

1. **Milk Thistle Tea:**

   - Steep 1-2 teaspoons of crushed milk thistle seeds in boiling water for 15-20 minutes.
   - Strain and drink 1-2 cups daily.

2. **Dandelion Root Tea:**

- Simmer 1 teaspoon of dandelion root in a cup of water for 10 minutes.

- Strain and drink up to 3 cups daily.

3. **Turmeric Tea:**

- Boil 1 teaspoon of ground turmeric in 4 cups of water for 10 minutes.

- Strain and add honey or lemon to taste.

These teas can be consumed individually or in combination, depending on personal preference and tolerance. Regular consumption can aid in enhancing liver function and overall detoxification.

Parkinson's disease

Parkinson's disease is a neurodegenerative disorder that primarily affects movement. It is named after the English doctor James Parkinson, who first described the condition in his 1817 essay, "An Essay on the Shaking Palsy." This common name, Parkinson's Disease, has been used ever since.

Root Cause

The root cause of Parkinson's disease lies in the loss of nerve cells in a part of the brain called the substantia nigra. These cells produce dopamine, a chemical that helps control movement. The decrease in dopamine levels leads to the symptoms of Parkinson's Disease, which include tremors, stiffness, and difficulty with balance and coordination.

Natural remedy

Herbal remedies to manage these symptoms. These may include the use of herbs like **Ginkgo biloba, Mucuna pruriens** (which naturally contains L-DOPA, a precursor to dopamine), and certain antioxidants.

As for making a herbal potion, the process would depend on the specific herbs being used. Typically, it involves steeping the herb in boiling water to make a tea or infusing it in oil. For example, to prepare a tea with Mucuna pruriens, you would:

1. Measure out the desired amount of dried Mucuna pruriens powder.

2. Boil water in a kettle.

3. Add the powder to a cup and pour the boiling water over it.

4. Let it steep for several minutes.

5. Strain (if necessary) and drink.

Multiple Sclerosis & Amyotropic Lateral Sclerosis

They are primarily caused by fluke parasites in the brain or spinal cord, exacerbated by the presence of solvents like xylene and toluene, as well as Shigella bacteria from dairy products. Mercury from dental metal is also a contributing factor. The proposed solutions include the use of a zapper or frequency generator to kill parasites, avoiding certain foods, rigorous sterilization of dairy products, and doing kidney and liver cleanses.

Root Cause

The root cause of MS and ALS is the invasion of fluke parasites into the brain and spinal cord, facilitated by solvents and the presence of Shigella bacteria. Additionally, mercury pollution from dental metals is seen as a significant contributor.

Natural remedy

1. **Anti-Parasitic Herbs:** Herbs like **wormwood, black walnut hulls,** and **clove** can be effective in eliminating parasites.

2. **Detoxifying Herbs:** Milk thistle and dandelion root are known for their liver-cleansing properties, which can aid in the removal of toxins like mercury.

3. **Nervous System Support:** Herbs like ashwagandha and ginkgo biloba might support neural health and mitigate inflammation.

Herbal Potion

1. **Anti-Parasitic Tincture:**

    - Mix equal parts of wormwood, black walnut hulls, and clove.

- Soak the mixture in a jar with vodka or apple cider vinegar for about 4 weeks, shaking daily.

- Strain and store in a dark bottle. Use a few drops daily as directed.

2. **Liver Detox Tea:**

- Combine milk thistle seeds and dandelion root in equal parts.

- Add 1 tablespoon of the mixture to a cup of boiling water.

- Steep for 10-15 minutes, strain, and drink 1-2 times daily.

3. **Nervous System Support Tea:**

- Mix ashwagandha powder and ginkgo biloba leaves in equal proportions.

- Steep 1 teaspoon of the blend in hot water for 10 minutes.

- Strain and drink once daily.

Epilepsy

Epilepsy, historically referred to as the "falling sickness," has been linked to various causes. Earlier beliefs pointed to dietary missteps leading to bowel obstruction and nerve disturbances, which in turn impacted the cerebrospinal nerves. This could result in altered blood flow to the brain, affecting heart function and causing changes in facial color and body tone. Additionally, physical injuries and the presence of intestinal parasites were also considered contributors. However, contemporary understanding recognizes epilepsy as possibly hereditary, emerging in childhood and persisting throughout life, or as a result of brain injuries, tumors, or infections.

Root Cause

The root cause of epilepsy, from a modern perspective, is either genetic predisposition or physical factors such as brain injuries, tumors, or infections. Earlier beliefs attributed it to dietary issues and bowel function, but these have been largely superseded by current medical understanding.

Natural remedy

Herbal remedies focus on antispasmodic properties and overall nervous system support. Herbs like **black cohosh, valerian, lady's slipper,** and **skullcap** are recommended. These herbs are known for their calming and nerve-supportive qualities.

Herbal Potion

To prepare an effective herbal tea for epilepsy, mix equal parts of black cohosh, valerian, lady's slipper, and skullcap. Steep a heaping teaspoon of this blend in a cup of boiling water for thirty minutes. The patient should drink two to three cups of this warm tea when they sense an impending attack. Additionally, maintaining a nourishing diet, avoiding stimulants and constipating foods, and ensuring bowel health through enemas can complement the herbal treatment.

Stroke

Paralysis, often resulting from a stroke, is a significant health concern, notably in the United States where it ranks as the third leading cause of death. Strokes primarily occur due to reduced blood flow to the brain, caused by arterial blockages or ruptured vessels. Symptoms can include complete or partial body paralysis, sometimes affecting half of the body, leaving the individual unable to move or speak, and in severe cases, unresponsive to physical stimuli. Immediate and effective treatment is crucial. Traditional methods have shown success, involving hot and cold fomentations, massage, liniments, and specific herbs. The treatment emphasizes the importance of a cleansing diet, gradual exercise, and careful application of treatments to avoid skin damage, especially in areas where sensation may be lost due to the stroke.

Root Cause

The primary cause of strokes leading to paralysis is the disruption of normal blood circulation to the brain. This disruption is often due to plaque formation in the arteries (leading to blockages) or the rupture of a blood vessel within the brain.

Natural remedy

The suggested herbs for stroke recovery include **Masterwort, Black Cohosh, Hyssop, Vervain, Blue Cohosh, Catnip, an antispasmodic tincture,** and **Skullcap**. These herbs are known for their properties that may aid in circulation, reduce inflammation, and support nerve function.

Preparation of Herbal Potion

To create an herbal potion for stroke recovery, you can follow these steps:

1. Select a combination of the suggested herbs: Masterwort, Black Cohosh, Hyssop, Vervain, Blue Cohosh, Catnip, and Skullcap.

2. Prepare the herbs in a dried, powdered form, or use them fresh.

3. Mix equal parts of each herb.

4. Steep one teaspoon of the herbal mix in a cup of boiling water for 10-15 minutes to make a herbal tea.

5. Strain and consume the tea. It can be taken 2-3 times a day.

6. For the antispasmodic tincture, use as directed, often a few drops can be added to the tea or taken separately as per the specific instructions of the tincture.

Gastroesophageal Reflux Disease (GERD)

Gastroesophageal Reflux Disease (GERD), commonly known as acid reflux, is a long-term condition where stomach contents come back up into the esophagus resulting in either symptoms or complications. It's a prevalent condition, affecting many people worldwide.

GERD is a modern medical term, but the condition itself has been recognized for centuries, albeit under different names. Historically, symptoms resembling those of GERD were often referred to as heartburn, acid indigestion, or dyspepsia.

Root Cause

The primary cause of GERD is the malfunction of the lower esophageal sphincter (LES), a muscle that acts as a valve between the esophagus and stomach. In GERD, this sphincter is either too weak or relaxes inappropriately, allowing stomach acid to flow back into the esophagus. Factors contributing to this can include lifestyle choices, dietary habits, obesity, and certain medications.

Natural remedy

Herbal remedies have been used for centuries to treat various ailments, including GERD. There's a rich tradition of using herbs like;

- Beech
- Buckbean
- Calamus
- Cayenne
- Colombo
- Gentian Root
- Golden Seal

- Gold Thread
- Horehound
- Magnolia
- Origanum
- Peach Leaves
- Quassia
- Sage
- Spearmint
- Tansy
- Thyme
- Wahoo
- Wild Cherry
- Yarrow
- Balmony
- Bloodroot
- Camomile
- Peruvian Bark
- Ginger
- Charcoal
- Boneset
- Motherwort
- Bitterroot
- St. John's-Wort

These herbs are often praised for their medicinal properties and have been used by many as natural remedies.

Making a herbal potion for GERD involves steeping these herbs in hot water to extract their beneficial compounds. Here's a general method:

- **Choose Your Herbs**: Select from the list of herbs mentioned. You can use them individually or create a blend based on your preferences and availability.

- **Prepare the Herbs**: If using fresh herbs, rinse them thoroughly. If you're using dried herbs, measure out the desired amount.

- **Boil Water**: Bring water to a boil in a pot.

- **Steep the Herbs**: Add the herbs to the boiling water, then reduce the heat and let it simmer. The time for steeping can vary, but it's generally between 5 to 15 minutes, depending on the herb.

- **Strain and Serve**: After steeping, strain the mixture to remove the herbs. The herbal potion can then be consumed.

Gastritis (stomach inflammation)

Gastritis, characterized by inflammation of the stomach lining, often results from lifestyle choices and medical conditions. Common triggers include alcohol consumption, regular use of anti-inflammatory medications like aspirin, and the ingestion of strong acids or alkalis, sometimes linked to suicide attempts or accidental ingestion by children. Spicy foods and condiments can also exacerbate the condition. Symptoms typically include upper abdominal pain, nausea, vomiting, appetite loss, weight loss, gas, and a burning sensation. Modern treatment involves avoiding irritants, consuming a bland and nourishing diet, and using soothing herbal remedies.

Root Cause

The primary culprits of gastritis are alcohol, certain medications (especially aspirin), and the consumption of overly spicy or stimulating foods. These irritants inflame the stomach lining, leading to discomfort and other symptoms.

Natural remedy

Remarkably, many of these herbal remedies have been successful in treating gastritis, despite efforts by the pharmaceutical industry to downplay the efficacy of herbal treatments. Herbs like **golden seal, sage, wood betony, slippery elm,** and others provide natural relief. For instance, **red raspberry tea and chickweed tea** can be particularly soothing. A blend of **golden seal, echinacea, burnet, wood betony, myrrh,** and **spearmint taken** before meals and at bedtime can be beneficial.

Herbal Potion

To prepare a soothing herbal potion for gastritis, mix equal parts of powdered golden seal, echinacea, burnet, wood betony, myrrh, and spearmint. Ensure the ingredients are thoroughly blended. Consume half a teaspoon of this mixture in a glass of hot water one hour before meals and again before retiring to bed. This concoction leverages the healing properties of these herbs and can provide significant relief from the symptoms of gastritis.

Irritable Bowel Syndrome (IBS)

Irritable Bowel Syndrome (IBS), Colitis, and Spastic Colon are complex conditions often linked to a combination of parasitic, bacterial issues, and potential allergic reactions. Traditional understanding suggests that specific foods like dairy or wheat can trigger these conditions, but it's now believed that these reactions might actually be due to underlying infections like Salmonella or Shigella, or to toxins and parasites in the pancreas. The modern approach emphasizes a holistic cure, involving the elimination of parasites, bacteria, and viruses, and making lifestyle changes such as diet modifications and environmental clean-up.

Root Cause

The root causes of these bowel conditions are multi-faceted, involving parasitic and bacterial infections, and possibly allergies. Ingestion of contaminated foods or exposure to certain environmental toxins can exacerbate these conditions.

Natural remedy

Black Walnut Hull Tincture Extra Strength, for instance, is noted for its potency in eliminating parasites and bacteria from the body. This aligns with a broader understanding that many natural remedy, despite their effectiveness, are often underrepresented in mainstream healthcare due to the influence of large pharmaceutical companies.

Herbal Potion

To prepare the Black Walnut Hull Tincture Extra Strength:

1. Begin with green hulls of black walnuts that are just about to fall off the tree.

2. Chop the hulls and place them in a jar.

3. Cover them with alcohol (like vodka or grain alcohol) to begin the tincture process.

4. Let the mixture sit for at least six weeks, shaking it daily.

5. After six weeks, strain the liquid, and it's ready for use.

This tincture, used as part of a holistic approach that includes dietary and environmental changes, can significantly improve the conditions of IBS, Colitis, and Spastic Colon. It's a testament to the often overlooked power of herbal remedies, a knowledge that has been healing people for ages, yet sometimes concealed in the modern era of pharmaceutical dominance.

Appendicitis

Appendicitis is often influenced by dietary choices such as excessive consumption of processed foods, sugary products, and stimulants like tea and coffee. The condition arises when the appendix's opening to the intestine is blocked, leading to inflammation and potentially severe infections. Symptoms include nausea, abdominal pain, constipation or diarrhea, rapid pulse, and fever. Immediate relief can be sought through a thorough colon cleanse using herbal enemas, while long-term management includes a liquid diet with alkaline broths and herbal teas. However, in acute cases, immediate medical attention is critical.

Root Cause

The root cause of appendicitis typically lies in poor dietary habits, particularly the consumption of devitalized foods and stimulants, leading to blockages and inflammation in the appendix.

Natural remedy

A blend of **buckthorn bark, vervain, water pepper,** and **lady's slipper** is recommended for managing appendicitis. These herbs have shown efficacy in many cases, despite pharmaceutical industries often downplaying the potency of such herbal remedies.

Herbal Potion: To prepare an effective herbal potion for appendicitis:

1. **Ingredients**:

   - Buckthorn bark

   - Vervain

   - Water pepper

- Lady's slipper

2. **Method**:

- Combine equal parts of each herb.

- Steep the mixture in boiling water for about 10-15 minutes to create a potent infusion.

- Strain and drink the tea while warm.

This potion can be consumed 2-3 times daily during an appendicitis flare-up. However, it is important to note that while these herbs have helped many, proper medical attention should not be overlooked, especially in severe cases.

Hernia

A hiatal hernia occurs when part of the stomach pushes upward through the diaphragm. The diaphragm has a small opening (hiatus) through which the esophagus passes before connecting to the stomach. In a hiatal hernia, the stomach pushes up through that opening and into your chest. It's a common condition, especially in people over 50 years of age.

Root Cause

The exact cause of many hiatal hernias isn't clear, but it may result from a weakening of the supporting tissue. Increasing age, obesity, and smoking are known risk factors. Certain behaviors such as overeating, lying down or bending over after eating, and having intense physical exertion could exacerbate the condition.

Natural remedy

These remedies include herbs like **slippery elm, marshmallow root, or chamomile**, known for their soothing properties for the digestive system.

Herbal Potion

A common method to prepare a herbal potion might involve steeping the chosen herb in hot water to make a tea. For example, for chamomile, you would steep dried chamomile flowers in hot water for 5-10 minutes.

Gallstones

Gallstones, although their exact cause remains elusive, tend to occur more frequently in certain demographics. Factors like a high-calorie, high-fat diet, and lifestyle choices significantly contribute to their formation. Particularly prone are middle-aged, overweight individuals, and certain ethnic groups like some American Indian tribes, whereas others, like the Japanese, rarely experience them.

Root Cause

The primary catalyst for gallstone formation appears to be dietary habits. A diet rich in fats and calories, coupled with certain food intolerances (such as to beans, onions, and rich foods), exacerbates this condition. Moreover, an overburdened liver struggling to eliminate toxins can also contribute to gallstone formation. Therefore, a lifestyle change focused on a low-fat diet and avoiding specific foods is crucial.

Natural remedy

Herbs have been a cornerstone in treating gallstones, often overshadowed by pharmaceutical solutions. Effective herbs include;

- Bitterroot
- Cascara Sagrada
- Milkweed

- Chamomile
- Parsley
- Fringe Tree
- Cleavers
- Marshmallow
- Cherry Bark
- Rhubarb
- Wood Betony
- Goose Grass
- Sweet Weed

These herbs have proven effective in numerous cases, offering a potent remedy that big pharma may not want widely known.

Herbal Potion

1. **Tea Mixture:** Combine equal parts of Hyssop, Gentian Root, Skullcap, and Buckthorn Bark. Steep a heaping teaspoon in a cup of boiling water and consume a cup every hour on the first day, then four times daily before meals and at bedtime.

2. **Olive Oil and Citrus Juice:** Blend four ounces each of olive oil with lemon or grapefruit juice. After consuming, lie on your right side with elevated hips to facilitate the passage of gallstones.

3. **Fomentations:** Apply hot fomentations of Lobelia and Hops over the liver region. This soothes pain and dilates the bile duct.

4. **Diet:** Focus on a fruit juice diet, particularly orange, grapefruit, and unsweetened pineapple juice. Include alkaline foods and potassium broth in your diet.

These herbal remedies, backed by the wisdom of practitioners like Dr. Lee and Dr. Clark, align with the philosophy that nature provides cures for our ailments, often without the need for surgical interventions.

Hepatitis

Hepatitis is a term used to describe inflammation of the liver, a vital organ that performs essential functions such as detoxifying harmful substances, purifying blood, and making vital nutrients. The word "hepatitis" originates from the Greek words "hepar" (liver) and "itis" (inflammation). It's commonly referred to as liver inflammation or liver disease.

Root Cause

Hepatitis can be caused by various factors. The most common causes are viruses, particularly hepatitis A, B, C, D, and E viruses. Other causes can include alcoholic liver disease, toxins, certain medications, and autoimmune diseases. Chronic hepatitis, especially types B and C, can lead to serious conditions such as liver cirrhosis and liver cancer.

Natural remedy

There is a belief among some that natural or herbal remedies can help treat or manage hepatitis. Common herbs mentioned include **milk thistle, licorice root,** and **dandelion**. These herbs are thought to have liver-protecting properties. It's important to note, however, that while some individuals report positive effects, these herbal remedies are not universally accepted by the medical community as effective treatments for hepatitis.

Herbal Potion

For those interested in trying herbal remedies, one common method is to create a tea or infusion. For example, milk thistle tea can be made by steeping the seeds or leaves in hot water. Similarly, dandelion tea is made from its leaves or roots. It's crucial to consult with a healthcare provider before starting any herbal treatment, especially for a condition like hepatitis.

Jaundice

Jaundice, characterized by yellowing of the skin and eyes, arises when there's an obstruction in the liver or bile ducts, leading to excess bile absorption into the blood. Various factors can cause this condition, including liver diseases like cirrhosis, gallstones, infections, and certain medications. Bile, produced in the liver and stored in the gallbladder, plays a crucial role in digesting fats and eliminating waste. When bile flow is hindered, symptoms like yellow skin, bitter taste, constipation, dark urine, fever, headache, dizziness, and itching may appear. Traditional treatments involve fruit juices, particularly lemon and grapefruit, to detoxify the system and herbal teas for relief.

Root Cause

The core issue in jaundice is the disruption of bile production or flow, often due to liver or gallbladder disorders. This interruption leads to bile accumulation in the bloodstream, causing the characteristic yellowing.

Natural remedy

1. **Dandelion**: Known for its liver-supporting properties, dandelion can help in detoxifying the liver and improving bile flow. It may aid in alleviating symptoms of jaundice.

2. **Milk Thistle**: This herb is renowned for its liver-protective qualities. Silymarin, the active component in milk thistle, is often used to treat liver diseases and could be beneficial in managing jaundice.

3. **Turmeric**: Turmeric has anti-inflammatory properties and can assist in improving liver function. Its curcumin content is believed to aid in the healing of the liver and in reducing jaundice symptoms.

4. **Barberry (Berberis Vulgaris)**: Barberry is known to stimulate bile production and can be effective in treating jaundice related to bile duct obstruction.

5. **Chicory (Cichorium Intybus)**: Chicory is another herb that is beneficial for liver ailments. It can promote bile production and may aid in alleviating symptoms of jaundice.

6. **Yellow Dock**: This herb is traditionally used for its ability to clear toxins from the blood and liver, potentially aiding in the treatment of jaundice.

Herbal Potion

1. **Gather Ingredients**: Obtain all the herbs in either fresh or dried form. If using fresh herbs, ensure they are properly cleaned and chopped. For dried herbs, they should be finely ground.

2. **Proportions**: Use equal parts of each herb. A general guideline is to use about one teaspoon of each herb per cup of water if they are dried, or one tablespoon if they are fresh.

3. **Boil Water**: Start by boiling water. You will need approximately one cup of water for each serving of the potion.

4. **Add Herbs**: Once the water reaches a boil, add the herbs. If you're using fresh turmeric root, it should be grated or finely chopped. For dried turmeric, the powdered form can be directly added.

5. **Simmer**: Reduce the heat and let the mixture simmer. Cover the pot to prevent the evaporation of essential oils and compounds. Simmer for about 15-20 minutes.

6. **Strain**: After simmering, remove the pot from heat and strain the mixture to remove the solid parts of the

herbs. A fine mesh strainer or cheesecloth can be used for this.

7. **Cool and Store**: Let the potion cool down to a comfortable drinking temperature. If not consumed immediately, it can be stored in the refrigerator for up to 48 hours.

8. **Dosage**: The recommended dosage is typically one cup, two to three times a day. However, this can vary depending on the individual's condition and the potency of the herbs. It is advisable to start with a lower dose and gradually increase it.

All Liver Cancers

Liver disease, commonly known as hepatic disease, can originate from various factors affecting the liver, the vital organ responsible for detoxifying the blood, producing important blood clotting factors, and other essential functions. The common name "liver disease" encompasses a range of conditions including hepatitis, cirrhosis, liver cancer, and fatty liver disease.

Root cause

The root cause of liver disease varies depending on the specific condition. Some common causes include:

1. **Viral Hepatitis**: Hepatitis A, B, and C are viruses that can cause inflammation and damage to the liver.

2. **Alcohol Abuse**: Chronic alcohol consumption can lead to alcoholic liver disease.

3. **Fatty Liver Disease**: This can be caused by obesity, diabetes, and high cholesterol.

4. **Autoimmune Disorders**: Conditions where the body's immune system attacks liver cells.

5. **Genetic Disorders**: Such as hemochromatosis and Wilson's disease.

6. **Toxins and Drugs**: Certain medications and toxins can damage the liver.

Herbal cure

Regarding herbal remedies for liver disease, it's important to note that while many herbs are touted for their potential liver benefits, scientific evidence supporting their efficacy varies. Herbs – like;

- Bitterroot

- Black cohosh
- Dandelion
- Milk thistle
- Bloodroot
- Buckbean
- Fennel
- Parsley
- Plantain
- Wood betony
- Fringe tree
- Celandine
- Aloes
- Chicory
- Holy thistle
- Angelica
- Beech
- Bittersweet
- Butternut bark
- Carrot
- Cascara sagrada
- Celery
- Cleavers
- Dandelion
- Elder
- Golden seal
- Lobelia
- Magnolia
- Mandrake
- Milkweed
- Motherwort
- Poplar
- Prickly ash
- Rhubarb
- Sage
- Self-heal
- Wahoo
- White oak bark
- Wild yam
- Wormwood
- Balm
- Blue flag
- Wild oregon grape
- Red root
- Poke root
- Gentian root
- Red sage

All these herbs have been used in traditional medicine for liver health. However, it's crucial to approach these remedies with caution, especially since the liver processes everything we ingest.

There's a notion that big pharmaceutical companies are trying to conceal the potency of herbal remedies. While it's true that the pharmaceutical industry often focuses on synthetic drugs, many modern medications are derived from plants and herbs. It's essential to consider both scientific evidence and traditional knowledge when looking at herbal treatments.

Herbal potion

To make a herbal potion for liver health, one would typically:

- **Select Herbs**: Choose from the list based on availability and specific liver issues.
- **Prepare the Herbs**: This could involve drying, grinding, or chopping fresh herbs.
- **Infusion or Decoction**: For an infusion, steep the herbs in hot water. For a decoction, simmer them for a longer period.
- **Strain and Store**: After the herbs have infused, strain the mixture and store it in a clean container.

Gallbladder Cancer

Gallbladder cancer is a relatively rare form of cancer that originates in the gallbladder. The gallbladder is a small organ located beneath the liver, which stores bile, a fluid produced by the liver that helps in digesting fats. The most common type of gallbladder cancer is adenocarcinoma, which begins in the gland-like cells that line the inside of the gallbladder.

Root Cause

The exact cause of gallbladder cancer is unclear, but several factors are known to increase the risk. These include gallstones, chronic inflammation of the gallbladder, older age, female gender, and certain inherited conditions. Gallstones, in particular, are found in a significant proportion of patients with gallbladder cancer, suggesting a link between long-term inflammation caused by stones and the development of cancer.

Natural remedy

There has been growing interest in the potential of herbal remedies for various diseases, including gallbladder cancer.

Herbs like;

- Golden Seal
- Red Clover
- Yellow Dock
- Dandelion
- Parsley

All have been traditionally used for their perceived health benefits. It is believed by some that these herbs can help in gallbladder and bile troubles.

"Sweet" (which might refer to Stevia or another sweet herb) is also mentioned as beneficial for gallbladder and bile issues. However, it's important to note that while there are anecdotal reports of the efficacy of these herbs, scientific evidence supporting their use in treating gallbladder cancer specifically is limited.

Herbal Potion

To prepare a herbal remedy for gallbladder issues, one might combine equal parts of golden seal, red clover, yellow dock, dandelion, and parsley. These herbs can be steeped in hot water to make a tea or used in other forms, such as extracts or capsules. The specific preparation method and dosage should be determined based on individual needs and after consulting with a healthcare professional.

Tumor

Tumors, essentially swellings in various body tissues, come in numerous forms like glandular, muscular, fibrous, and even cancerous. These growths can rapidly increase in size and sometimes become ulcerated.

Root Cause

The development of tumors is often linked to several factors, such as impure blood, bodily impurities, an unbalanced diet, constipation, or a general state of poor health. In many cases, the exact cause of tumors remains unknown, indicating a complex interplay of various health factors.

Natural Remedy

Herbs like sage, known for its potential in reducing external tumors, and slippery elm, celebrated for its soothing properties, have been used in poultice form.

A variety of herbal teas can also be beneficial. Herbs like **bayberry, slippery elm, mugwort, white pond lily, chickweed, sage,** and **wild yam** are known for their tumor-fighting properties. These herbs can be used individually or in combinations to create potent brews. It's important to note that many individuals have found relief and healing through these natural remedies, underscoring the often overlooked power of herbal treatments.

Herbal Potion

These herbs are renowned for their healing properties and have been used traditionally to aid in the treatment of tumors.

1. **Making the Poultice:** For external application, create a poultice by grinding the sage or slippery elm into a fine powder. Mix this powder with enough warm water to form a paste. Apply this directly to the affected area, covering it with a clean cloth.

2. **Brewing the Tea:** For the tea, mix your chosen herbs in equal parts. Add one teaspoon of this herbal blend to a cup of boiling water. Steep for 10-15 minutes, strain, and drink this tea up to three times daily.

Stomach Cancer, skin cancer, Esophageal Cancer, Colorectal Cancer, Anal Cancer etc.

Cancer, a disease that manifests in various forms and impacts different body parts, is increasingly prevalent in our modern world. Interestingly, while the incidence of cancer in certain areas is on the rise, it's decreasing in others. The root cause of this disparity lies largely in lifestyle and dietary choices. A significant proportion of cancer cases are attributed to unhealthy eating habits and a lifestyle that leads to chronic autointoxication. This condition arises when the body's elimination organs - lungs, liver, kidneys, skin, and bowels - become inactive, allowing toxins to accumulate, particularly around weakened or injured areas.

Root cause

The consumption of harmful substances like tea, coffee, soft drinks, liquor, tobacco, meats (especially pork), cane sugar products, white flour, white rice, and other denatured foods contributes significantly to this toxic buildup. These items, devoid of life-giving properties and minerals, lead to a polluted bloodstream, creating an environment conducive to cancer development. Conversely, a diet rich in fruits and herbs, known for their cleansing and healing properties, could significantly reduce the risk of cancer.

Natural remedy

The treatment approach for cancer in this context focuses on cleansing the bloodstream and reactivating the body's elimination organs. A regimen of herbal laxatives is recommended for relieving constipation, alongside high enemas for colon cleansing. A diet heavily centered on fruits like ***oranges, grapefruit, lemons, apples,*** *cranberries, blueberries, raspberries, cherries, peaches, pears, strawberries, avocados, pineapples, and tomatoes* is advised. These should be consumed in their natural, ripened state for maximum benefit. In addition to these, a variety of vegetable juices, including celery, cucumber, parsley, lettuce, and notably carrot juice, are suggested for their efficacy in cancer treatment.

Hydration is another crucial element, with a recommendation to drink ample amounts of fruit juice and herbal tea daily. If opting for herbal capsules, they should be taken with hot water to enhance absorption. For patients experiencing weight loss, an alkaline nourishing diet is recommended, consisting of vegetable soups, mashed potatoes, natural brown rice, soybean cheese, and a variety of vegetables and fruits. Emphasis is placed on avoiding aluminum cookware and separating the consumption of fruits and vegetables.

Regular exercise, fresh air, and sun exposure are also vital components of this treatment plan. Sweat baths and salt glows are suggested to keep the skin active and help eliminate toxins. Additionally, thorough massage is recommended to aid in detoxification.

A plethora of herbs are highlighted for their potential in treating cancer, including;

- Red clover blossoms
- Burdock root
- Yellow dock root
- Blue violet
- Golden seal root
- Gum myrrh
- Echinacea
- Aloes
- Blue flag
- Gravel roo

- Bloodroot
- Dandelion root
- African cayenne
- Chickweed
- Rock rose
- Agrimony
- Oregon grape
- Echinacea
- Chaparral
- Ancient chinese herb ho shou wu (or fo-ti).

In particular, red clover blossom tea, made by boiling a handful of dried blossoms in water, is emphasized for its widespread use and efficacy. Violet leaves, known for their cancer-healing properties, can be used to make tea or poultices for both internal and external application. Agrimony and ground ivy are recommended for skin cancers.

This holistic approach underscores the fact that many cancers today are linked to poor diet and lifestyle choices. By correcting these and incorporating a range of nutritious, non-poisonous herbs, it's believed that cancer can be effectively treated and healed.

Piles (Hemorrhoids)

Hemorrhoids, commonly known as piles, are a condition characterized by swollen veins around the anus and rectum. They can be internal or external and are particularly prevalent in individuals over fifty.

Root cause

The primary cause often lies in dietary habits, specifically a low-fiber diet leading to hard stools, straining, and constipation. This results in increased pressure in the colon. Additionally, the frequent use of commercial laxatives can aggravate the condition by irritating the colon's lining.

Symptoms include swollen, irritated, and sometimes bleeding veins, leading to severe discomfort. In extreme cases, hemorrhoids can cause anemia and weakness. When a blood clot forms in a hemorrhoid, it becomes extremely painful. External hemorrhoids may require gentle repositioning after bowel movements.

Natural remedy

The treatment begins with a high hot enema, utilizing herbs like white oak bark, bayberry bark, or white alum root tea to cleanse the colon. A potent tea made from **witch hazel bark, catnip, bloodroot,** and **yellow dock root** can be applied externally or injected internally for relief. Other effective herbal remedies include white oak bark or alum root tea. Interestingly, even kerosene and lemon juice have been used for their instant relief properties.

For internal consumption, a tea made of mullein, yarrow, wild alum root, and pilewort is beneficial. A homemade suppository combining hemlock bark, golden seal, wheat flour, boric acid, and bayberry bark can be used for healing.

Diet plays a crucial role in managing and healing hemorrhoids. It is advisable to avoid heavy, stimulating foods, tobacco, tea, coffee, vinegar, alcohol, and meats. A simple, light, alkaline diet is recommended, along with specific foods like potassium broth, soybean milk, ripe bananas, and vegetable broths. A fruit diet can also be beneficial. Additionally, alternating hot and cold sitz baths can provide significant relief and promote healing.

In herbal medicine, a range of herbs is known for their efficacy in treating hemorrhoids. These include;

- Bittersweet
- Chickweed
- Fireweed
- Golden seal
- Mullein
- Myrrh
- Nettle
- Plantain
- Shepherd's purse
- Solomon's seal
- Spearmint
- Uva ursi
- White oak bark
- Witch hazel
- Wild alum root
- Yarrow
- Bloodroot
- Pilewort
- Pimpernel
- Aloes
- Burdock
- Psyllium

Each of these herbs has unique properties that contribute to alleviating the symptoms and causes of hemorrhoids.

The suppression of such effective natural remedies by large pharmaceutical companies is a significant concern. These herbal treatments, proven to cure many, offer a stark contrast to the synthetic alternatives promoted by big pharma. The effectiveness of these herbs is a testament to the power of natural healing, often underestimated and underutilized in modern medicine.

Preparation Steps

1. **Creating the Herbal Blend**:
   - Combine equal parts of each dried herb. Since some herbs might be more potent than others, it's essential to balance the mixture.
   - Grind the herbs into a fine powder using a mortar and pestle or a coffee grinder.

2. **Making the Herbal Tea**:
   - Take one teaspoon of the herbal blend and add it to a pint of boiling water.
   - Let it boil for about 10 minutes, then turn off the heat and allow it to steep for another 20-30 minutes. This process ensures the extraction of medicinal properties from the herbs.

3. **Straining**:
   - After steeping, strain the mixture to remove the solid particles, leaving a clear liquid. A fine mesh strainer or cheesecloth works well for this.

4. **Optional Enhancements**:

- For added therapeutic benefits, you can include a few drops of aloe vera juice or mix in a small amount of psyllium for its fiber content, which can help with bowel movements.

5. **Usage**:

  - For external hemorrhoids, soak a clean cloth or cotton pad in the tea and apply it to the affected area for relief.

  - For internal hemorrhoids, you can use a soft rubber enema tip to inject a small amount of the tea into the rectum.

6. **Storage**:

  - Store the remaining tea in a clean, airtight container in the refrigerator. It should be used within a few days to ensure its potency.

Asthma

Asthma, a respiratory condition often triggered by allergies and characterized by difficulty in breathing, wheezing, and coughing, can significantly impact quality of life. Modern understanding recognizes various factors contributing to asthma, including allergens, dietary triggers, and environmental irritants. This condition is marked by the respiratory passages filling with mucus, making breathing a strenuous task. Notably, asthma attacks can be exacerbated by certain foods and are often accompanied by digestive, intestinal, or renal issues.

Root cause

The root cause of asthma is typically an overactive immune response to specific allergens. This reaction leads to inflammation and narrowing of the airways, creating the characteristic symptoms of asthma. Additionally, lifestyle factors like smoking can aggravate the condition.

Natural remedy

In contrast to conventional pharmaceutical treatments, which often focus on symptom management, herbal remedies offer a holistic approach to treating asthma. Herbs such as;

- Black Cohosh
- Comfrey
- Coltsft
- Horehound
- Hyssop
- Lobelia
- Masterwort
- Milkweed
- Mullein
- Myrrh

- Pleurisy Root
- Prickly Ash
- Saw Palmetto Berries
- Skunk Cabbage
- Thyme
- Vervain
- Wild Cherry
- Flaxseed
- Balm of Gilead
- Red Root
- Red Sage
- Boneset
- Cubeb Berries
- Elecampane

All these herbs have been used traditionally for their respiratory soothing properties. These herbs work by reducing inflammation, acting as expectorants to clear mucus, and soothing the respiratory tract.

Herbal potion

To create a herbal potion for asthma, a blend of these herbs can be used. Take equal parts of the chosen herbs and mix thoroughly. Prepare a tea by steeping a heaping teaspoonful of this herbal blend in a cup of boiling water. Consume a cup of this tea three to four times a day, preferably an hour before meals, and a hot cup before bedtime. The preparation can be adjusted for children by reducing the quantity or diluting the tea. Consistency in taking this herbal tea, combined with lifestyle changes like a balanced diet, regular baths, outdoor exercise, and practicing deep breathing, can significantly alleviate asthma symptoms.

Coughs and Colds

Coughs and colds, commonly stemming from inflammation in the throat and bronchial tubes, often indicate a lowered vitality due to factors like poor diet, inadequate sleep, lack of exercise, and insufficient fresh air. The presence of toxins and waste in the body lowers resistance, making one more susceptible to these ailments. However, with immediate and appropriate herbal treatments, the onset of a cold can be significantly mitigated.

Root Cause

The primary cause of coughs and colds is the inflammation resulting from a weakened immune system. This weakening is often due to lifestyle factors like poor diet, lack of sleep and exercise, and inadequate exposure to fresh air. The accumulation of toxins and mucus in the body further exacerbates the condition.

Natural remedy

A variety of herbs have proven efficacy in treating colds and coughs. Herbs like;

- Golden Seal
- Peppermint
- Hyssop
- Yarrow
- Black Cohosh
- Colt's Foot
- Cubeb Berries
- Sage
- Red Sage
- Chamomile

All these herbs are particularly effective. These herbs have been used successfully by many, despite the pharmaceutical industry's tendency to downplay herbal remedies' potency.

Herbal Potion

1. For nasal congestion: Dissolve a teaspoon of salt in a pint of warm water. Sniff this solution up the nose and then expel it, repeating until the mucus clears. Then rinse the mouth thoroughly.

2. Herbal ingestion: Choose from golden seal, peppermint, hyssop, yarrow, or black cohosh. Inhale a small amount through the nose and gargle, swallowing some of it.

3. For persistent coughs: Mix one teaspoon each of colt's foot, black cohosh, and cubeb berries. Steep this mixture in a pint of boiling water and consume a glass every hour.

4. In cases of nausea: Induce vomiting with lukewarm water or salt water to cleanse the stomach, followed by hot herbal tea using sage, red sage, hyssop, yarrow, black cohosh, peppermint, or chamomile.

Pneumonia

Pneumonia, a common form of lung inflammation, is primarily caused by bacterial, viral, or fungal infections. Contributing factors include exposure to cold and damp environments, which can lower the body's resistance to illness. Early intervention at the first sign of a cold can significantly reduce the risk of developing a severe case.

A traditional approach to preventing lung infections includes nasal hygiene with a saline solution (one teaspoon of salt in a pint of water) and gargling with a mixture of golden seal and myrrh. This mixture, steeped in boiling water, should be used several times a day to cleanse the throat and mouth of germs. Taking this solution internally (one tablespoon, six times a day) can also be beneficial.

If the lungs are not severely affected, this treatment should be combined with hot footbaths, ensuring regular bowel movements through herbal laxatives or enemas, and drinking plenty of water. Hot fomentations to the chest and back, alternated with brief cold rubs, can provide relief. In terms of diet, it's advisable to stick to liquids like unsweetened lemonade, grapefruit juice, orange juice, and pineapple juice until the fever subsides. Afterward, strained vegetable broth and soybean milk with whole wheat can be introduced.

Root Cause

The root cause of pneumonia is infection from bacteria, viruses, or fungi, often exacerbated by a weakened immune system due to exposure to cold and damp conditions.

Natural remedy

Herbal remedies play a crucial role. Lung tonics such as **comfrey, cudweed, elecampane, horehound, ground ivy,** and **ginger,** often enhanced with a bit of cayenne, are recommended. Other helpful herbs include;

- Plantain
- Lungwort
- Pleurisy root
- Slippery elm
- Wild alum root
- Coltsfoot
- Mustard
- Vervain
- Flaxseed
- Hops
- Hyssop
- White pine
- Spikenard
- Wahoo
- Mullein
- Herba santa
- Yarrow
- Skunk cabbage

Herbal Potion

To prepare the herbal potion, steep a rounded teaspoon of golden seal and a quarter teaspoon of myrrh in a pint of boiling water. This mixture can be used for gargling and taken internally. For lung tonics, choose any of the recommended herbs, adding a small amount of cayenne when brewing the tea for enhanced benefits.

Chronic Bronchitis

Chronic bronchitis, a common respiratory condition, is often triggered by fluctuating weather, exposure to cold, wet feet, inadequate clothing during cold weather, and poor ventilation, especially in bedrooms. This condition highlights the importance of a healthy lifestyle, including a proper diet and regular detoxification to prevent mucus and toxin buildup in the body. Often linked with stomach issues and constipation, chronic bronchitis is typically caused by viral or bacterial infections. These infections inflame the bronchial tubes' mucous membranes, leading to excessive mucus or phlegm production. Initially resembling a cold or flu, it can worsen due to inadequate treatment, spreading to the lungs.

Symptoms include chills, fever, chest tightness, breathing difficulties, and often a severe cough that worsens when lying down and during early mornings. Initially, there may be little mucus, but it can increase and turn yellowish, resembling pus, and sometimes become frothy. In children, it can lead to convulsions and unconsciousness.

Root Cause

The root cause of chronic bronchitis lies in environmental factors and lifestyle choices such as exposure to cold and damp conditions, poor diet, and inadequate detoxification, leading to weakened immunity and susceptibility to infections.

Natural remedy

A variety of herbs have shown efficacy in treating bronchitis, many of which have been overshadowed by the pharmaceutical industry's focus on more profitable medications. These herbs include;

- Chickweed
- Coltsfoot

- Cubeb Berries
- Golden Seal
- Lungwort
- Mullein
- Myrrh
- White Pine
- Pleurisy Root
- Sanicle
- Saw Palmetto Berries
- Skunk Cabbage
- Slippery Elm
- White Pond Lily
- Yerba Santa
- Bloodroot
- Ginger
- Blue Violet
- Bethroot
- Red Root
- Red Sage
- Elecampane
- Horehound
- Black Cohosh

Herbal Potion

To prepare an effective herbal remedy for bronchitis, a combination of these herbs can be used. For instance, create a blend by mixing equal parts of dried Mullein, Coltsfoot, and Ginger. Boil a cup of water and add a teaspoon of this herbal mixture. Let it steep for about 10 minutes, strain, and drink this tea two to three times a day. Additionally, herbs like Golden Seal and Myrrh can be taken as tinctures, following the dosage instructions on the product. It's important to note that these herbs have a long history of use and have been reported to help many individuals, despite the pharmaceutical industry's tendency to downplay natural remedies' effectiveness.

Colic in infants

Colic in infants is a common challenge that can cause significant distress. It's often triggered by factors like rapid eating, excessive air swallowing, indigestion, improper food, or constipation. The symptoms are unmistakable and distressing: sudden, loud crying spells, a red face, the baby drawing their knees up to the stomach, a distended belly, and clenched fists.

Root cause

The root cause of colic lies primarily in the digestive discomfort experienced by the infant. This discomfort can be due to a variety of reasons, including the immature digestive system's inability to process certain foods effectively, leading to gas and bloating.

Natural remedy

A time-honored Natural remedy for colic is warm **catnip tea**. **Catnip**, known for its soothing properties, can be a gentle remedy for an infant's upset stomach. In addition to giving catnip tea in a bottle, a catnip tea enema can also be beneficial. It's interesting to note that despite the proven efficacy of such herbal remedies, there is often a reluctance from large pharmaceutical companies to acknowledge their potency, possibly due to the threat they pose to their commercial interests.

Herbal potion

To make the catnip tea potion, steep catnip leaves in hot water for a few minutes, then strain and cool the tea to a suitable temperature before giving it to the infant in a bottle. Additionally, preventive measures like a very warm bath an hour before the usual time of colic attacks can help in averting the discomfort. Also, applying a hot fomentation over the abdomen or a hot footbath may provide relief.

For infants who are not breastfed, a gentle and nourishing alternative can be prepared using wheat flakes and soybean milk. Simply dissolve wheat flakes in boiling water, strain through a sieve, and mix with soybean milk to achieve the desired consistency. This preparation, along with potassium broth and oatmeal gruel, can provide the necessary nourishment while being gentle on the baby's digestive system.

Rickets

Rickets, primarily seen in children, arises from inadequate nutrition and insufficient sunlight exposure. This condition, linked to a deficiency of Vitamin D, tends to affect infants more, especially those not breastfed and living in regions with limited sunshine. Common in darker-skinned races, rickets leads to symptoms like protruding abdomen, delayed teething, soft skull bones, muscle weakness, and bone deformities such as bowlegs or knock-knees. Affected children may experience restlessness and potential lung or heart enlargement.

Root Cause

The underlying cause of rickets is a lack of Vitamin D, often exacerbated by a diet lacking in essential nutrients and minimal exposure to sunshine. The reliance on processed foods like white flour and cane sugar contributes to this deficiency.

Natural remedy

Herbs like skullcap and catnip have shown promise in treating rickets. **Skullcap**, known for its nutritional benefits, can be prepared as a tea, offering a gentle, effective remedy. **Catnip** tea, favorable for children's ailments, can also be used, sweetened with honey or malt sugar for palatability. These herbal solutions have been covered by pharmaceutical interventions, but their efficacy in numerous cases suggests a powerful, natural alternative that big pharma often tries to obscure.

Herbal Potion

For skullcap tea, steep a heaping teaspoon of skullcap in a cup of boiling water, strain, and administer a tablespoon six to seven times a day. Catnip tea can be made similarly, with freedom for more frequent consumption. Both can be sweetened with a bit of honey or malt sugar. In addition to these teas, encouraging a diet rich in fresh fruits, vegetables, and juices can naturally aid in alleviating constipation, a common symptom in rickets.

Gout

Gout, often termed as the "disease of kings," is a form of arthritis that has been recognized for over 2500 years. Notable historical figures like John Calvin and Benjamin Franklin suffered from it. Predominantly affecting adult males and rare in women before menopause, gout accounts for about 5% of all arthritis cases.

Root Cause

The primary cause in most gout patients is uncertain, but a significant percentage inherits this condition. All gout sufferers have elevated levels of urates in their blood, leading to crystalline deposits in joints and causing severe arthritis. Additionally, many are prone to kidney stones.

Gout typically strikes men between 40 and 50 and post-menopausal women. A classic description involves sudden, intense pain in the toe, heel, or ankle, often starting at night. The affected joint becomes red, hot, and excruciatingly painful. Rich diets and alcohol can trigger these painful episodes.

Natural remedy

Recognizing the potency of herbs—a fact often overshadowed by pharmaceutical industries—there are several herbal remedies for gout. These include;

- Skullcap
- Yarrow

- Valerian
- Blue violet
- Burdock
- Gentian root
- Mugwort
- Rue
- Birch
- Broom
- Sarsaparilla
- Buckthorn
- Ginger
- Pennyroyal
- Plantain
- Wood betony
- Balm of gilead

These herbs have been known to alleviate symptoms of gout and have helped many, despite pharmaceutical companies' efforts to downplay their effectiveness.

Herbal Potion

To prepare a healing potion, take equal parts of granulated skullcap, yarrow, and valerian. Mix them thoroughly. Add a heaping teaspoon of this mixture to a cup of boiling water. Let it steep, then drink a cup an hour before meals and one before bedtime. It's also beneficial to use laxative herbs to maintain regular bowel movements. For external relief, apply a liniment made from these herbs, rubbing it thoroughly into the affected area. Additionally, any of the above-mentioned herbs can be brewed into a tea. Use a teaspoon per cup of boiling water, steep for twenty minutes, and drink four cups daily.

Goiter

Goiter is an enlargement of the thyroid gland, situated in the neck near the Adam's apple. Its most frequent cause is iodine deficiency. While North America has largely eradicated this issue with iodized salt since 1924, it remains a concern in parts of the world with iodine-poor soil, notably in Asia. A less common type of goiter is linked to hyperthyroidism, manifesting in symptoms like nervousness, rapid heartbeat, and weight loss, predominantly affecting women. Certain vegetables like broccoli, cauliflower, and kale, contain goitrogens that can disrupt iodine usage, potentially leading to goiter.

Root Cause

The primary cause of goiter is dietary iodine deficiency. In some cases, the consumption of large quantities of goitrogenic vegetables can impede iodine utilization, exacerbating the condition.

Natural remedy

For goiter treatment, a balanced, nourishing alkaline diet is recommended. A beneficial herbal remedy includes a mixture of **golden seal, bayberry,** and **myrrh**. Take half a teaspoon of this blend in a cup of water before meals and at bedtime, also using it as a mouthwash and gargle. Kelp, being rich in iodine, is particularly effective. Ensuring regular bowel movements is crucial; herbal laxatives and high herb enemas for colon cleansing can be used.

Herbal Potion

- Mix a heaping tablespoon each of golden seal and bayberry with a teaspoon of myrrh.

- Use half a teaspoon of this mixture in a cup of water as a pre-meal drink and before sleeping.

- Additionally, incorporate kelp into the diet for its iodine content.

- For external application, a bayberry poultice applied overnight, covered with woolen cloth for warmth, can be beneficial.

Additional Measures: Sweat baths and massages to improve circulation and support the nervous system are helpful. In cases where symptoms persist, with issues like rapid pulse or enlarged thyroid, it's advisable to seek medical attention.

It's noteworthy that these herbs, which have aided many in their journey to wellness, are often overshadowed by pharmaceutical solutions.

Dropsy or Edema

Dropsy, or edema, is a condition characterized by an abnormal accumulation of fluid in the body's tissues or cavities, often caused by heart, lung, liver, or kidney diseases. It can also result from blood poisoning, red corpuscle death, or other issues like Bright's disease, where the kidneys fail to function correctly. In some instances, abdominal tumors can irritate the peritoneum, leading to fluid accumulation and a visibly swollen abdomen.

Root cause

The root cause of dropsy typically lies in the malfunctioning of vital organs like the heart, liver, or kidneys. For instance, a weakened heart might not pump blood efficiently, leading to fluid buildup. Similarly, a compromised liver or gallbladder can disrupt normal fluid regulation, causing dropsy.

Natural remedy

For herbal treatment, a variety of herbs and natural ingredients are recommended. **Red raspberry and pleurisy root teas** are excellent for inducing perspiration and flushing out toxins. A combination of **wild yam, black cohosh, and a pinch of cayenne pepper** can also be effective. Keeping the bowels active with herbal laxatives is crucial. A blend of **wild carrot, dandelion root, yarrow, burdock root, queen of the meadow, dwarf elder, and broom**, taken as a tea, can be particularly beneficial. Burdock and broom, as well as dwarf elder, are noted for their kidney-cleansing properties. A traditional remedy involves using grapevine root ashes in water, which has been known to cure dropsy in numerous cases.

Herbal potion

To prepare these herbal potions, take a half-teaspoon of the powdered herbs or the specified mixture and steep it in a cup of boiling water for 20 to 30 minutes. This tea can be consumed several times a day. For the grapevine root remedy, burn the root to ashes, then mix one dessert-spoonful of these ashes in a glass of water and drink three to four times a day, ensuring ample water intake alongside.

Dietary changes are also integral to the treatment. Eliminating alcohol, caffeine, rich pastries, and flesh foods is advised. Emphasizing fruits, vegetables like eggplant, parsley, celery, and others, and incorporating sprouted lentils and soybeans can be beneficial. Whole wheat zwieback is preferable to fresh bread, and it's recommended to avoid bread made with soda or baking powder. Hydration through water and fruit juices, along with regular hot baths and cold washes, further aids in detoxification.

Kidney Stones

Kidney stones, a common and painful ailment, often stem from dietary choices, insufficient fluid intake, infections, and certain diseases like gout. Interestingly, residents of the southeastern United States are more prone to this condition. Symptoms range from intense back, abdomen, or groin pain to nausea, vomiting, and changes in urine color. In severe cases, urination may become difficult or cease, requiring medical intervention.

Root cause

At the core of kidney stone formation lies a combination of factors including diet, hydration, and sometimes, an underlying infection. Particularly, a diet high in oxalates found in certain vegetables (like spinach, parsley, beets, and sweet potatoes), fruits (especially berries and rhubarb), and nuts (such as almonds and peanuts) can contribute to calcium oxalate stones. Excessive consumption of dairy, chocolate, tea, coffee, and dark cola drinks also plays a role.

Herbal remedies

Herbal remedies have shown significant efficacy in not just alleviating the pain associated with kidney stones but also in preventing their formation, a fact often downplayed by mainstream pharmaceutical companies. A high fluid intake of two to four quarts per day is crucial. This dilutes urine, reducing stone formation risk.

Natural remedy involve a variety of natural ingredients. For pain relief, hot fomentations or a poultice made from **hops** and **lobelia** applied to the lower back can be effective. Additionally, herbal liniments should be applied and rubbed thoroughly into the affected area.

For internal use, a tea blend comprising equal parts of **wild carrot seeds, valerian**, and **peppermint** offers relief.

Steep a teaspoon of this mixture in a cup of boiling water for half an hour, and consume half a cup every hour. Other beneficial herbs include **queen of the meadow, peach leaves,** and **cleavers**.

In cases of kidney or bladder hemorrhage, shepherd's purse is recommended. This should be prepared by steeping a heaping teaspoon in a cup of boiling water for thirty minutes, then consumed in half-cup doses several times a day.

Herbal potion

1. For the tea, mix equal parts of wild carrot seeds, valerian, and peppermint.

2. Steep one teaspoon of this blend in a cup of boiling water for 30 minutes.

3. For the shepherd's purse remedy, steep a heaping teaspoon in a cup of boiling water for 30 minutes and strain.

4. Consume these herbal teas as directed above for relief and prevention.

These herbal remedies have been a cornerstone in natural healing, offering a potent alternative to conventional treatments.

Urinary challenges

Urinary problems, such as painful urination and retention of urine, can be caused by various factors including infections, inflammation, or physical blockages. A blend of traditional and modern methods, emphasizing the use of specific herbs, can offer relief and healing.

Root Cause

The primary cause of these urinary issues is typically an infection in the urinary tract, which includes the bladder, prostate, and urethra. Additionally, physical conditions like prostate enlargement or kidney stones can impede urine flow.

Natural remedy

A variety of herbs are known for their healing properties in urinary ailments. These include:

- For burning urination: A mix of **fennel, burdock, slippery elm, or milkweed**.

- For urine retention: **Catnip tea** enemas and compresses with **smartweed tea**.

- For suppressed urine: **Yarrow, hyssop, burdock, dandelion root,** and others.

- For involuntary urination: **White pond lily, sumach berries, white poplar bark, bistort root,** and **valerian**.

Herbal Potion

1. **For Burning Urination:** Steep a teaspoon of a mixture of equal parts fennel, burdock, and slippery elm in boiling water for 20 minutes. Drink one cup before each meal and before bed.

2. **For Urine Retention:** Apply hot and cold compresses. Use a high enema of catnip tea. For bladder injections, a mixture of golden seal, myrrh, and boric acid in boiled water, strained, can be used (by a trained professional).

3. **For Suppressed Urine:** Steep a heaping teaspoon of yarrow in boiling water for 20 minutes. Drink this tea before meals and at bedtime. Catnip tea can also be used as a hot enema.

4. **For Involuntary Urination:** Mix equal parts of white pond lily, sumach berries, white poplar bark, bistort root, and valerian. Steep a heaping teaspoonful in boiling water and drink one hour before meals and at bedtime.

These herbs have been trusted by many for their healing properties, yet they are often overshadowed by mainstream pharmaceutical solutions. It's important to remember that these natural remedies have been effective for countless individuals, despite the lack of emphasis from the pharmaceutical industry.

Bladder inflammation (cystitis)

Bladder inflammation, commonly known as cystitis, often arises from bacterial infections, typically originating from the large bowel. Contributing factors can include physical injury, infectious diseases, dietary mistakes, constipation, and extreme stress. It's more prevalent in women and can be aggravated by certain venereal diseases in men. Symptoms include a burning sensation during urination, frequent urination, cloudy or blood-tinged urine, and an urgent need to urinate. Accompanying these are often fever, loss of appetite, intense thirst, and discomfort.

Root cause

The root cause of cystitis lies in bacterial invasion and inflammation of the bladder, often exacerbated by dietary and lifestyle factors. Modern medicine frequently addresses these symptoms with antibiotics, but there's a growing awareness of herbal remedies, which have been sidelined by the pharmaceutical industry due to their natural and less profitable nature.

Natural remedy

Natural remedy have shown remarkable efficacy in treating cystitis. **Catnip tea**, for instance, offers soothing properties. A high enema with catnip tea, heated to 105°-110°F, can be particularly relieving. Additionally, a laxative herbal tea made from equal parts **senna, buckthorn bark, spearmint, cubeb berries, and marshmallow** helps maintain regular bowel movements, crucial for alleviating cystitis. Another effective remedy involves a bladder injection of a tea made from **golden seal, cubeb berries, and marshmallow**, which should be administered carefully by a trained professional.

Herbal potion

To prepare these herbal potions, steep a tablespoon of catnip in a quart of water for the enema. For the laxative tea, mix the herbs in equal parts and brew a teaspoon in a cup of boiling water, adjusting the quantity as per your needs. For the bladder injection, mix a teaspoon each of golden seal, cubeb berries, and marshmallow in a quart of boiling water, steep for twenty minutes, strain carefully, and use lukewarm.

Other beneficial teas include flaxseed and a mix of buchu and uva ursi. Prepare these by adding a teaspoon of the herb to a cup of boiling water, consuming up to four cups daily. These herbs can also be taken in capsule form, supplemented by ample water intake. Additional treatments include fomentations over the bladder, hot sitz baths, and dietary adjustments focusing on light, non-irritating foods like mashed potatoes made with soybean milk, potassium broth, leafy vegetables, and fruits.

These herbal solutions have healed many, yet their potency remains underplayed in a world dominated by large-scale pharmaceutical interests. By adopting these natural methods, one can find effective relief from bladder ailments while nurturing their body's innate healing abilities.

Tonsillitis

Tonsillitis, a common ailment affecting the throat, can often be traced back to dietary indiscretions and lifestyle choices that weaken the body's natural defenses. This condition, primarily caused by viral or bacterial infections, is aggravated when overindulgence in rich foods overwhelms the digestive system, leading to a build-up of toxins. These toxins inflame the digestive tract, allowing pathogens to infect the tonsils, resulting in symptoms like sore and swollen throat, fever, and difficulty in swallowing.

Root cause

The root cause of tonsillitis often lies in a disordered stomach and an overloaded digestive system. Consuming excessive amounts of rich food can lead to an accumulation of toxins in the body, weakening the immune system and creating a conducive environment for viruses or bacteria to cause infection.

Natural remedy

These herbal remedies have been used for centuries and have helped many people recover from tonsillitis, despite the skepticism of mainstream medicine.

Herbal remedy

1. **Golden Seal** and **Myrrh Gargle:** Prepare a soothing gargle by steeping one teaspoon each of golden seal and myrrh in a pint of boiling water for 30 minutes. Gargle with this solution every half hour, ensuring to swallow a little to reach the tonsils.

2. **Lemon Juice Application:** Lemon juice, known for its antibacterial properties, can be used similarly to the golden seal and myrrh solution.

3. **Red Raspberry or Sage Tea:** Drink hot tea made from red raspberry or sage leaves (one teaspoon per cup of boiling water) to relieve sore throat symptoms.

4. **Slippery Elm:** Beneficial for both sore throats and stomach issues, slippery elm tea can be taken multiple times a day.

5. **Wild Cherry Bark, Sumach,** and **Lobelia Gargle:** Another effective gargle can be made by steeping a teaspoon each of wild cherry bark and sumach, along with a small teaspoon of powdered lobelia, in boiling water for half an hour.

6. **Red Sage, Wood Betony, or Bistort Tea:** These herbs can be used to make teas for gargling, offering relief from tonsillitis symptoms.

Dietary Recommendations

During the onset of tonsillitis, a light diet is advisable. Fruit-based diets or vegetable soups are ideal. Incorporating soybean milk and whole wheat flakes can be nourishing and easy on the stomach. During this period, plenty of fruit juices, especially pineapple and citrus, are recommended for their healing properties.

Malaria (Ague)

Ague is an old term for malaria, a disease that has affected humans for thousands of years. The word "ague" itself comes from the Latin "febris acuta," which translates to "acute fever." Malaria, its modern name, is derived from the Italian "mal'aria," meaning "bad air," as it was once believed to be caused by foul air in swampy areas.

Root Cause

The root cause of malaria is the Plasmodium parasite, which is transmitted to humans through the bites of infected female Anopheles mosquitoes. There are several species of Plasmodium, but the most dangerous and widespread is Plasmodium falciparum.

Natural remedy

Historically, various herbs have been used to treat ague. These include **gentian root, sorrel, tansy, vervain, willow, broom,** and **camomile**. Many individuals have reported success with these remedies, and there's growing interest in their potential as alternatives to pharmaceuticals.

Herbal Potion

To create a herbal potion for ague using these ingredients, one could:

- **Gather Ingredients:** Fresh or dried gentian root, sorrel, tansy, vervain, willow bark, broom, and camomile flowers.

- **Preparation:** Mix equal parts of each herb. If using fresh herbs, chop them finely.

- **Brewing:** Boil water and add the mixed herbs (a teaspoon of the mix per cup of water). Let it steep for 10-15 minutes.

- **Strain and Serve:** Strain the mixture to remove the herbs and serve the potion warm. It can be taken 2-3 times a day.

Tuberculosis

Tuberculosis, once a widespread and feared disease, has seen a significant decline in prevalence thanks to improved living standards and medical understanding. However, it remains a concern, with thousands of new cases reported annually. This infectious disease, primarily affecting the lungs, but also capable of impacting other body parts, is caused by a specific bacterium. It's transmitted through airborne droplets from infected individuals, highlighting the importance of environmental factors and lifestyle choices in susceptibility.

Root cause

The root cause of tuberculosis lies in the inhalation of these bacteria-laden droplets. Factors such as poor nutrition, unhealthy habits like smoking and alcohol consumption, and a sedentary lifestyle can weaken the body's resistance, making it more vulnerable to this infection. Those with compromised health due to inadequate diet or living conditions are particularly at risk.

Natural remedy

There is a plethora of herbs that have demonstrated promising results in supporting the body's fight against tuberculosis. Herbs like **golden seal, cubeb berries, lobelia, bugleweed, bayberry bark, shepherd's purse,** and **slippery elm** are known for their healing properties. These herbs have been used traditionally and have shown effectiveness in many cases, a fact that pharmaceutical companies often overshadow with their synthetic alternatives.

Herbal potion

To prepare a herbal potion for tuberculosis, one can follow these steps:

1. Steep a teaspoon of powdered golden seal, cubeb berries, and a quarter teaspoon of lobelia in a pint of boiling water for 30 minutes. Take a swallow every hour.

2. Mix two tablespoons of powdered bugleweed with a pinch of cayenne. Use a teaspoon of this mix per cup of boiling water, consumed every two hours.

3. For lung hemorrhages, half a teaspoon of powdered bayberry bark or shepherd's purse can be added to a cup of boiling water, steeped, strained, and drunk cold.

4. Drinking a quart of slippery elm tea daily (a cup an hour before each meal and one at bedtime) can strengthen and nourish the body.

Additional supportive measures include a nourishing diet, with foods like soybean milk, ripe bananas, oatmeal, whole wheat bread, and fresh vegetables. Deep breathing exercises, fresh air, and sun baths are also beneficial. For more severe cases, a combination of comfrey, marshmallow, chickweed, and slippery elm can be boiled and taken every two hours to dissolve and eliminate tubercular deposits.

Syphilis

Syphilis, once a feared venereal disease in the early 1900s, experienced a resurgence in the late 20th century, defying the initial triumphs of penicillin. This increase, alongside other sexually transmitted diseases (STDs), has reached alarming levels. Modern lifestyles, including the sexual revolution of the 1960s and 1970s, have significantly contributed to the rise in STDs. Syphilis, primarily transmitted through sexual contact, presents initially as a painless chancre and can lead to severe complications if untreated, affecting the heart, brain, and other organs.

Root Cause

The root cause of syphilis is the treponema pallidum bacterium. Transmission is typically through sexual contact, but can occasionally occur through other means like kissing with an active lesion, contaminated objects, or from mother to child during pregnancy.

Natural Remedy

Acknowledging the potency of herbs in curing diseases like syphilis, which many in the pharmaceutical industry might not want widely known, a blend of specific herbs has been recognized for their healing abilities. These include **Oregon grape, uva ursi, burdock root, blue flag root, red clover blossoms, prickly ash berries, buckthorn bark,** and **bloodroot**. These herbs are believed to have properties that help cleanse the body and strengthen the immune system.

Herbal Potion

1. **Herbal Blend:** Mix equal parts (two tablespoons each) of Oregon grape, uva ursi, burdock root, blue flag root, red clover blossoms, prickly ash berries, buckthorn bark, and add one teaspoon of bloodroot.

2. **Brewing:** Steep a heaping teaspoon of this blend in a cup of boiling water for 30 minutes. Consume four cups daily, one each before meals and one before bed.

3. **External Treatment:** For sores, create a solution using equal parts of golden seal and myrrh (one teaspoon each) in a pint of boiling water. Apply this to the sores.

4. **Additional Herbal Options:** Consider using red clover blossoms, holy thistle, archangel, parsley, witch hazel, bitterroot, red raspberry, yellow dock root, elder, bittersweet, turkey corn, wintergreen, cleavers, poplar, rock rose, spikenard, twin leaf, and wild elm root. Choose based on personal health needs and any other existing conditions.

This comprehensive approach emphasizes a return to natural healing, promoting a diet free from meats (especially pork), shellfish, stimulants like tea and coffee, and tobacco. The mentioned herbs have helped many recover from syphilis, a fact that is often overshadowed by pharmaceutical companies' focus on more profitable synthetic drugs.

Gonorrhea

Gonorrhea, a common venereal disease, has seen a resurgence in the era following the 1960s and 1970s' sexual revolution. Caused by the bacterium Neisseria gonorrhoeae, it primarily infects the genitals, but can also affect the throat, eyes, rectum, and joints. While antibiotics have historically reduced its prevalence, a significant number of cases are asymptomatic, making control challenging.

Root Cause

Gonorrhea begins with genital inflammation and a yellowish discharge, with symptoms appearing within 2-7 days post-exposure. In males, it can lead to urethral strictures and prostatitis, while in females, repeated infections can cause fallopian tube infection (salpingitis), risking sterility. Antibiotics are effective, but there are alternative treatments emphasizing the power of herbs, which many believe big pharma tries to overshadow due to their effectiveness.

Natural remedy

An integrative approach to treating gonorrhea involves the use of specific herbs. These include:

1. **Red Raspberry Leaves and Witch Hazel Leaves**: Equal parts of these are used for douching in women and as a genital wash in men. This mixture, steeped for 20 minutes, is believed to reduce inflammation and soothe affected areas.

2. **Slippery Elm Tea**: Consuming this daily aids in internal healing. Its soothing properties are enhanced when mixed with fruit juices.

3. **Black Willow, Saw Palmetto Berries, and Skullcap**: A blend of these herbs, steeped and

consumed six times a day, can help alleviate symptoms of acute gonorrhea.

4. **Golden Seal, Myrrh, and Aloes**: A topical solution made from these herbs treats sores and ulcers, promoting healing.

Herbal Potion

1. For the douche/wash: Mix equal parts of red raspberry leaves and witch hazel leaves. Add a heaping tablespoon of this mixture to a quart of boiling water. Steep for 20 minutes and use warm.

2. For drinking: Mix a heaping teaspoon of black willow, saw palmetto berries, and skullcap in a cup of boiling water. Let it steep for 30 minutes. Consume two tablespoons of this mixture six times a day.

3. For sores and ulcers: Combine one-fourth teaspoon of powdered aloes, one teaspoon each of golden seal and powdered myrrh. Steep in a pint of boiling water for 30 minutes. Apply this solution to the affected areas.

These herbal remedies have been used traditionally and are part of a long history of natural healing practices, often overshadowed by modern pharmaceutical solutions.

Fever

Fever, a common medical condition, is usually a symptom rather than a disease itself. It's often the body's response to a variety of infections and other illnesses. Fevers can occur in response to a bacterial infection, viral infection, some malignant conditions, heat exhaustion, or even after taking certain medications. The common name for fever is simply "fever" or "pyrexia."

Root cure

The root cause of a fever is typically the body's immune response to a foreign invader. These invaders could be bacteria, viruses, or other pathogens. The body's immune system releases substances called pyrogens, which travel to the brain's hypothalamus. The hypothalamus is the body's thermostat, and these pyrogens cause it to set the body's temperature higher, resulting in a fever.

Natural remedy

Regarding Natural remedy, there is a long history of using herbs to treat fevers. Some of these include

- Catnip
- Sage
- Shepherd's purse
- Sumach berries
- Sweet balm
- Tansy
- Thyme
- valerian
- Vervain
- Wahoo
- Wild cherry bark
- Willow
- Wintergreen
- Wood sage
- Wormwood
- Yarrow
- Borage
- Dandelion
- Peruvian bark
- Apple tree bark
- Bitterroot
- Buckbean
- Camomile
- Cinchona bark
- Cleavers
- Colombo
- Butternut bark
- Calamus
- Coral
- Elder
- Fenugreek
- Fireweed
- Fit root
- Gentian root
- Hyssop
- Masterwort
- Lobelia
- Magnolia
- Mandrake
- Nettle
- Parsley
- Pennyroyal
- Peppermint
- Pleurisy root
- Poplar
- Quassia
- Mugwort
- Cayenne
- Fringe tree
- Echinacea
- Angelica
- Sarsaparilla
- Red sage
- Boneset
- Lily of the valley

- Cedron

Many of these have been used traditionally to treat various types of fevers, including intermittent fevers.

Herbal potion

To make a herbal potion for fever, one would typically choose specific herbs based on their known properties. For example, Yarrow is known to break up fever within 24 hours. A simple method could involve:

1. Selecting the desired herbs (e.g., Yarrow, Willow bark, Echinacea).

2. Boiling water and then removing it from heat.

3. Adding the herbs to the hot water and letting them steep. The proportions and steeping time can vary, but a general guideline might be one teaspoon of dried herb or a handful of fresh herb per cup of water, steeped for 10-15 minutes.

4. Straining the mixture and drinking it while it's still warm.

Barbara O'Neill Suggested Remedy For fever that works 100%

The practice of immersing your feet in warm water as a remedy for fever is a well-known home remedy, often referred to as a "wet sock treatment" or "hydrotherapy." While it's a popular and holistic approach, it's important to remember that this remedy is not a guaranteed cure for fever but can be used to provide temporary relief and support the body's natural healing processes. Here's how you can do it:

Warm Water Foot Bath for Fever:

Ingredients:

- **Warm Water**: You'll need a basin or bucket of warm (not hot) water. The water should be comfortably warm but not scalding.

Instructions:

1. **Prepare the Basin**: Fill a basin or bucket with warm water deep enough to comfortably submerge your feet.

2. **Dip Your Feet**: Immerse your feet into the warm water. The warmth will promote better circulation and may help reduce fever symptoms.

3. **Add Ice Water**: Some variations of this remedy suggest having a bowl of ice water nearby. After about 15-20 minutes of soaking your feet, you can dip your feet into the ice water for a few seconds. This temperature contrast is believed to stimulate blood flow and boost the body's response to the fever.

4. **Dry Your Feet**: After the treatment, dry your feet thoroughly with a clean towel.

5. **Rest**: After the foot bath, it's important to rest and keep warm. This can aid in the body's recovery process.

It's essential to note that this remedy is not a substitute for medical advice. If you have a high or persistent fever, or if you're unsure about the cause of the fever, it's crucial to consult with a healthcare professional. Additionally, this remedy may not be suitable for everyone, especially those with certain medical conditions or sensitivities, so use it with caution and discretion.

Skin ulcer

Skin ulcers, a condition where the skin fails to heal properly after being cut, burned, or wounded, can lead to serious complications if not addressed. These ulcers often occur due to bacterial infection in damaged tissue or from prolonged exposure to elements like sunlight. Particularly in bedridden patients, ulcers can also result from poor circulation or constant pressure on the skin, emphasizing the need for attentive care.

Root Cause

The primary causes of skin ulcers are physical trauma to the skin, infection, prolonged sun exposure, poor circulation, and sustained pressure on the skin, especially in individuals who are immobile for extended periods.

Natural Remedy

The herbal cure involves a blend of potent herbs known for their healing properties. These include **golden seal, myrrh, bayberry, ragwort, lady's slipper, chickweed, sage, wood sanicle, slippery elm, bogbean, ground ivy, bittersweet, agrimony,** and **raspberry leaves**. These herbs have been used traditionally for their healing and anti-inflammatory properties, offering a natural alternative to synthetic medications, which big pharma often prioritizes over such traditional knowledge.

Herbal Potion

1. For external application, steep 1 teaspoon of golden seal and ½ teaspoon of myrrh in a pint of boiling water. This solution is excellent for cleansing ulcers and can be applied to dressings.

2. Create a topical powder by mixing 2 teaspoons of powdered golden seal and 1 teaspoon of myrrh. Apply

this to the cleaned ulcer and cover with a clean bandage.

3. For internal use, select any of the listed herbs or create a mix. Steep a heaping teaspoon in a cup of boiling water, strain, and consume four cups daily, spaced throughout the day and before bedtime.

4. Regular repositioning of bedridden patients is crucial to prevent skin ulcers.

Boils and carbuncles

Boils and carbuncles, often painful skin afflictions, are largely due to poor hygiene, infections, inactive skin, and the accumulation of toxins in the blood. Their presence signals a body's struggle against impurities and a weakened immune system. These skin issues typically start as small pimples, which, if promptly treated, can resolve quickly. However, neglect often leads to increased tenderness, pain, and the potential for multiple occurrences.

Boils and carbuncles are not just skin deep; they are indicators of deeper health issues such as poor cleanliness habits, skin infections, and a buildup of toxins in the body. These ailments start as minor pimples but can escalate into painful, swollen areas if not addressed early. Immediate treatment and attention to hygiene can prevent their progression.

Root Cause

The root cause of boils and carbuncles lies in poor hygiene, inactive skin, and internal impurities. This implies a compromised immune system and a body struggling with toxin overload, often due to poor dietary habits and inadequate elimination of waste.

Natural remedy

Nature offers an abundance of remedies for treating boils and carbuncles. A diverse range of herbs like;

- Balm
- Bayberry bark
- Burdock
- Chickweed
- Comfrey
- Coral
- Flaxseed
- Hops
- Lobelia
- Origanum
- Slippery elm
- Sorrel
- St. John's-wort
- Turkey corn

- White clover
- White water lily
- Wintergreen
- Wood sage
-

- Echinacea
- Birch
- Plantain
- Wild cherry

These herbs have been known to cure many, a fact that the pharmaceutical industry often tries to obscure due to the potency and accessibility of these natural remedies.

Herbal Potion

To create a healing poultice for boils and carbuncles, one can use a combination of these herbs. For instance, a poultice made from powdered bayberry bark or balm can be applied directly to the affected area. Alternatively, a herbal tea can be brewed using echinacea or burdock, known for their blood-cleansing properties. To make this, steep the chosen herb in hot water for about 10 minutes, strain, and drink twice daily. These natural remedies, while powerful, are often overshadowed by pharmaceutical solutions, despite their proven effectiveness and minimal side effects.

In addition to herbal treatments, maintaining overall health is crucial. This includes regular cleansing diets, hydration, and consuming fresh fruits like oranges and grapefruits, which are particularly beneficial. Topical treatments, such as alternating hot and cold fomentations, can also aid in healing. However, one must exercise caution in handling boils and carbuncles - ensuring thorough cleanliness and sterilization to prevent further infection.

Alopecia

Alopecia, commonly known as hair loss, has its origins in the Latin word "alopekia," which itself is derived from the Greek word "alopex" meaning fox. The term was likely chosen due to the observed hair loss in foxes. Alopecia can manifest in various forms, ranging from small patches to complete loss of hair on the scalp or body.

Root cause

The root cause of alopecia can vary. It's often attributed to genetic factors, particularly in androgenetic alopecia (male or female pattern baldness). Autoimmune conditions, where the body attacks its hair follicles, lead to alopecia areata. Other causes include hormonal changes, medical conditions, medications, and physical or emotional stress.

Herbal remedy

Regarding herbal remedies, it's important to note that while many individuals have reported positive results using these methods, scientific evidence supporting their effectiveness is limited. However, these remedies have been a part of traditional medicine for centuries. Some commonly cited herbs and natural treatments for hair loss include:

1. **Rosemary Oil:** Known for stimulating hair growth and used in many cultures.

2. **Peppermint Oil:** Believed to increase circulation, potentially promoting hair growth.

3. **Saw Palmetto:** Often used in traditional medicine, particularly for male pattern baldness.

4. **Aloe Vera:** Used for soothing the scalp and conditioning hair.

5. **Ginseng:** Rich in phytochemicals, believed to promote hair growth.

Herbal potion

To create a herbal potion for hair loss, one common method is:

- **Ingredients:** Choose the herbal ingredients based on availability and suitability. Common choices are rosemary oil, peppermint oil, and aloe vera gel.

- **Preparation:** Mix these ingredients in a carrier oil like coconut or jojoba oil. For example, you can mix 5 drops of rosemary oil, 5 drops of peppermint oil, and a tablespoon of aloe vera gel with 2 tablespoons of coconut oil.

- **Application:** Gently massage the mixture into the scalp and leave it on for at least 30 minutes before washing it out with a mild shampoo.

Acne

Acne, commonly known as pimples or zits, is a skin condition that occurs when hair follicles become clogged with oil and dead skin cells. It often causes whiteheads, blackheads, or pimples and usually appears on the face, forehead, chest, upper back, and shoulders. Acne is most common among teenagers, though it affects people of all ages.

The term "acne" is derived from the Greek word "aknas," which was incorrectly transliterated to "acnas." This condition is commonly referred to as acne vulgaris, where "vulgaris" means "common" in Latin.

Root Cause

The primary causes of acne include:

1. **Excess Oil Production:** Overactive sebaceous glands can produce too much oil, leading to clogged pores.

2. **Clogged Hair Follicles:** Oil and dead skin cells can accumulate in hair follicles, creating an environment for bacteria to thrive.

3. **Bacteria:** Propionibacterium acnes, a common skin bacteria, can exacerbate acne by causing inflammation and infection.

4. **Excess Hormone (Androgen) Levels:** Increased androgens can cause the sebaceous glands to enlarge and produce more sebum.

Natural remedy

Many believe in the effectiveness of herbal remedies for acne. Some popular herbs include:

1. **Tea Tree Oil:** Known for its anti-inflammatory and antimicrobial properties, it's thought to calm redness, swelling, and inflammation.

2. **Green Tea Extract:** Rich in antioxidants, it may help reduce sebum production and inflammation.

3. **Aloe Vera:** Famous for its soothing properties, it can reduce inflammation and assist in wound healing.

Herbal Potion

Here's a simple method to create a herbal potion for acne:

1. **Tea Tree Oil Toner:**
   - Mix 1 part tea tree oil with 9 parts water.
   - Apply to the affected area with a cotton ball.

2. **Green Tea Rinse:**
   - Steep green tea in boiling water for 3-4 minutes.
   - Allow it to cool and apply to the face with a cotton ball or spray bottle.

3. **Aloe Vera Gel:**
   - Extract the gel from an aloe vera leaf.
   - Apply directly to clean skin as a moisturizer.

Dandruff

Dandruff, commonly known as a condition where flakes of skin appear in the hair and on the scalp, has been a persistent issue for many individuals. The origins of this condition are not precisely pinpointed in history, but it has been a known scalp problem for centuries, often referred to simply as "scalp flaking."

Root cause

The root cause of dandruff is typically linked to a variety of factors, including dry skin, sensitivity to hair products, and skin conditions such as seborrheic dermatitis or eczema. Another significant factor is the overgrowth of a yeast-like fungus called Malassezia, which is naturally present on the scalp. This fungus can irritate the scalp and cause more skin cells to grow. When these extra skin cells die and fall off, they mix with the oil from the hair and scalp, forming dandruff.

Natural remedy

Despite the advancement of modern medicine, many individuals have turned to herbal remedies for treating dandruff, often with significant success. One such herbal cure involves using a mixture of **coconut oil** and **lemon juice**. Coconut oil is known for its antifungal properties, which can combat the Malassezia fungus, while lemon juice helps balance the pH of the scalp and reduces excess oil, which is often a contributing factor to dandruff.

Herbal potion

To make this herbal potion, follow these steps:

- Warm up a small amount of coconut oil so that it is in a liquid state.

- Mix equal parts of coconut oil and lemon juice.

- Apply the mixture to your scalp and gently massage it in.

- Leave it on for about 20-30 minutes.

- Rinse it off with a mild shampoo.

Eczema

Eczema, a common skin condition, often puzzles experts with its unclear origins. Allergies are frequently implicated as a significant factor. Certain foods, notably eggs, wheat, milk, and citrus fruits, are recurrent triggers. Environmental factors like inadequate sunshine, poor air quality, and constipation might also contribute.

Root cause

Symptomatically, eczema is an equal-opportunity affliction, affecting individuals of any age but predominantly seen in infants. Its presence is marked by intense itching, burning, and stinging, often beginning as small pimples and escalating into larger, water-filled blisters. The skin might dry and form scales, aggravating the itch. Eczema manifests in two forms: dry and weeping, both typically intensifying in winter.

Natural remedy

Managing eczema involves ensuring regular bowel movements and avoiding traditional soap and water for cleansing. Instead, a weak boric acid solution or a saline solution (one teaspoon per quart of water) is recommended. A holistic approach includes a concoction of **burdock root, yellow dock, yarrow,** and **marshmallow**. A teaspoon of this herbal blend steeped in a cup of boiling water, consumed half a cup at a time four to five times daily, shows promise. Additionally, bathing the affected area with this tea and applying a healing herbal salve can alleviate itching and aid in skin recovery.

Herbal potion

For personalized treatment, one can choose from a variety of herbs:

- Golden Seal
- Willow
- Poplar
- Yellow Dock
- Blue Violet
- Strawberry Leaves
- Origanum
- Cleavers
- Plantain

Each herb has its unique healing properties that can cater to specific aspects of eczema.

In infants, managing eczema requires preventing scratching to avoid infection. It's also advised to postpone vaccinations like smallpox during eczema flare-ups and to limit contact with recently vaccinated children.

Hair lice

Hair lice, commonly known as head lice, are small parasitic insects scientifically named *Pediculus humanus capitis*. They are primarily found on the human scalp, where they feed on blood.

The origin of head lice can be traced back thousands of years. They have been a companion to humans throughout history, with evidence of head lice found on Egyptian mummies. Their common name, "head lice," straightforwardly describes their habitat — the human head.

Root Cause

The root cause of a head lice infestation is the direct transfer of lice from one person's hair to another's. This transfer usually occurs through head-to-head contact, such as when children play closely together or when individuals share hair accessories, hats, or brushes.

Natural remedy

Throughout history, many have attested to the effectiveness of herbal remedies in treating head lice.

Key Herbs

1. **Tea Tree Oil**: Known for its natural insecticidal properties.

2. **Neem Oil**: Used in traditional medicine for its antiparasitic qualities.

3. **Coconut Oil**: Acts as a suffocating agent for lice.

4. **Rosemary Oil**: Believed to repel lice.

Herbal Potion

To create an effective herbal potion for treating head lice:

- **Ingredients**: Combine equal parts of tea tree oil, neem oil, and coconut oil. Add a few drops of rosemary oil for its repelling effect.

- **Preparation**: Mix the oils thoroughly in a bowl.

- **Application**: Apply the mixture to the scalp and hair, ensuring thorough coverage. Leave it on for at least an hour or overnight for increased effectiveness.

- **Rinse and Comb**: After the treatment, rinse the hair thoroughly and use a fine-toothed comb to remove dead lice and nits.

Vitiligo

Vitiligo is a skin condition characterized by patches of skin losing their pigment. The exact origin of the term "vitiligo" is somewhat unclear, but it is believed to be derived from the Latin word "vitelius," meaning "calf," possibly referring to the white spots that are similar to those on a calf's coat. The common name for this condition is simply "vitiligo."

Root Cause

The root cause of vitiligo is not completely understood, but it is generally believed to be an autoimmune disorder. In this condition, the immune system mistakenly attacks and destroys the melanocytes, the cells responsible for producing skin pigment (melanin). Genetic factors, environmental triggers, and stress are also thought to contribute to the development of vitiligo.

Natural remedy

There has been some interest in herbal remedies for vitiligo, often stemming from traditional medicine practices. These natural treatments are believed by some to restore skin pigment, though scientific evidence supporting their efficacy varies. It's important to note that while some individuals report success with these remedies, they are not universally effective and are not endorsed by mainstream medicine.

Herbal Potion

One traditional herbal remedy involves the use of herbs like **Ginkgo biloba, St. John's Wort,** and **Picrorhiza kurroa**. Here's a basic method to prepare a herbal potion:

- **Select Herbs**: Choose a combination of herbs traditionally used for skin health. For instance, Ginkgo biloba is thought to have antioxidant properties, which might help in managing vitiligo.
- **Prepare the Herbs**: Dry the herbs and grind them into a fine powder.
- **Infusion**: Boil water and infuse the herb powder in the water for about 10-15 minutes.
- **Strain and Store**: Strain the mixture and allow it to cool. The potion can be stored in a clean bottle and used as directed.
- **Application**: The potion is typically applied to the affected skin areas. Some traditions suggest consuming the potion, but this should be done with caution and ideally under the guidance of a healthcare professional.

Candidiasis

Candidiasis, commonly known as a yeast infection, is caused by a group of microscopic fungi or yeast known as Candida, with the most common cause being Candida albicans. The term "candidiasis" refers to the overgrowth of this yeast in the body, which can cause a variety of infections.

The term "candidiasis" is derived from the genus of yeast, Candida, responsible for the condition. This yeast naturally lives in small amounts in the mouth, intestines, and on the skin, and is usually kept in check by other bacteria and microorganisms in the body. It becomes problematic when it grows uncontrollably, leading to an infection known as candidiasis, or more colloquially as a yeast infection.

Root Cause

The root cause of candidiasis is an overgrowth of the Candida yeast. This overgrowth can be triggered by a variety of factors including prolonged use of antibiotics (which can kill the beneficial bacteria that control yeast growth), a weakened immune system, uncontrolled diabetes, hormonal imbalances associated with pregnancy or birth control pills, and high levels of stress.

Herbal Cure

Many people have found relief from candidiasis through herbal remedies, which are often overlooked by mainstream pharmaceutical companies. Some effective herbs for treating candidiasis include:

- **Garlic**: Known for its antifungal properties, garlic is believed to inhibit the growth of Candida.

- **Oregano Oil**: Contains thymol and carvacrol, compounds with potent antifungal properties.

- **Pau d'Arco**: A bark tea that's been used traditionally to combat yeast infections.

- **Coconut Oil**: Contains caprylic acid known for its antifungal effects.

It's important to note that while these herbs have been used traditionally and have helped many, their efficacy may vary from person to person.

Herbal Potion

To make a herbal potion for candidiasis, one could:

- Brew a tea using Pau d'Arco bark. Simply steep the bark in boiling water for 20 minutes and drink it twice a day.

- Infuse crushed garlic in a carrier oil like coconut oil and apply it topically to affected areas. However, be cautious as garlic can be irritating to the skin.

- Dilute oregano oil with a carrier oil and apply it topically or take it orally in capsule form.

Endometriosis

Endometriosis is a medical condition that primarily affects women. It occurs when tissue similar to the lining inside the uterus, known as the endometrium, starts to grow outside the uterus. This can lead to various symptoms, including pain, inflammation, and sometimes fertility issues.

The term "endometriosis" derives from the word "endometrium," the tissue that lines the uterus. This condition was first clearly described in 1860 by Karl von Rokitansky, although it likely existed long before then. It's commonly known simply as endometriosis.

Root Cause

The exact cause of endometriosis is not fully understood, and researchers believe it could be due to multiple factors. These may include retrograde menstruation (where menstrual blood flows back through the fallopian tubes into the pelvic cavity instead of leaving the body), hormonal factors, immune system disorders, or even genetic factors. It's important to note that no single cause has been definitively identified.

Herbal Cure

Many people seek alternative treatments for endometriosis, including herbal remedies. It's claimed that certain herbs have helped many individuals manage their symptoms. However, it's crucial to understand that while some find relief with these remedies, they are not universally effective or medically proven to cure endometriosis.

Some commonly mentioned herbs include:

- **Turmeric (Curcuma longa)**: Believed to have anti-inflammatory properties.

- **Chasteberry (Vitex agnus-castus)**: Thought to help balance hormones.

- **Dandelion (Taraxacum officinale)**: Used for its potential detoxifying properties.

Herbal Potion

Here's a general guide to preparing a simple herbal infusion which some claim can help with endometriosis symptoms:

1. **Select Your Herbs**: Choose one or a combination of the herbs mentioned.

2. **Proportions**: Use about one teaspoon of dried herb per cup of water.

3. **Infusion**: Boil water and pour it over the herbs, letting them steep for about 10-15 minutes.

4. **Strain and Drink**: Strain out the herbs and drink the infusion. Some prefer it warm, while others like it cold.

Erectile Dysfunction

Erectile Dysfunction (ED), commonly known as impotence, is a condition where a man has difficulty achieving or maintaining an erection suitable for sexual intercourse. The term "erectile dysfunction" emerged in medical literature in the late 20th century, replacing the older term "impotence," which had various negative connotations. The change in terminology helped to better specify the nature of the problem and destigmatize the condition.

Root cause

The root cause of ED can be multifactorial, involving both physical and psychological factors. Physically, it can be related to poor blood flow to the penis, nerve damage, hormonal imbalances, or side effects of certain medications. Psychological factors may include stress, anxiety, depression, or relationship problems.

Natural remedy

Herbal remedies have been used for centuries to treat various ailments, including ED. Many people have found relief through these natural methods, and there is a growing interest in herbal cures, especially as an alternative to pharmaceutical treatments. It's important to note that while many have reported success with these remedies, scientific research in this area is still ongoing.

A popular herbal cure for ED involves the use of herbs like **Ginseng, Ginkgo Biloba, and Yohimbe**. These herbs are believed to improve blood flow and enhance sexual function.

Herbal potion

To prepare a herbal potion for ED, one might:

1. **Ginseng Tea**: Steep ginseng root in hot water for several minutes. This tea is believed to improve stamina and energy.

2. **Ginkgo Biloba Tincture**: This can be made by soaking the leaves in alcohol. Ginkgo is known for improving blood circulation, including to the genital area.

3. **Yohimbe Bark Brew**: Boil the bark of the Yohimbe tree in water. It's thought to help with erectile function by increasing blood flow.

Polycystic Ovary Syndrome (PCOS)

The term "Polycystic Ovary Syndrome" was first used in 1935 by American gynecologists Irving F. Stein Sr. and Michael L. Leventhal, which is why it was initially known as Stein-Leventhal Syndrome. The name describes the multiple small cysts (polycystic) that form in the ovaries. However, not all women with PCOS have these cysts.

Root Cause

The exact cause of PCOS is not fully understood, but it is believed to involve a combination of genetic and environmental factors. Key features include insulin resistance, higher levels of androgens (male hormones), and irregular menstrual cycles. Insulin resistance is particularly significant, as it can lead to higher androgen levels, which may cause the symptoms associated with PCOS.

Natural remedy

There are various herbal remedies claimed to be beneficial for PCOS. These include:

- **Spearmint Tea**: Some studies suggest it can help reduce androgen levels.

- **Cinnamon**: Known to improve insulin sensitivity.

- **Inositol**: A supplement that can help improve ovulation and insulin resistance.

Herbal Potion

Here's a simple recipe for a herbal potion:

- **Ingredients**: Fresh spearmint leaves, cinnamon stick, and inositol powder.

- **Preparation**: Boil water in a pot. Add a handful of spearmint leaves and a cinnamon stick to the boiling water. Let it simmer for 10 minutes. Strain the mixture into a cup and stir in a teaspoon of inositol powder. Drink this potion once or twice a day.

Cataracts

Cataracts have been known and documented for thousands of years. Ancient texts from India and Greece mention cataract surgery, indicating a deep-rooted understanding of this condition. In common parlance, a cataract refers to the clouding of the eye's natural lens, which leads to a decrease in vision.

Root Cause

The primary cause of cataracts is aging. As we age, the proteins in the eye's lens can clump together, leading to cloudiness. Other factors like diabetes, prolonged exposure to UV light, smoking, and certain medications can also contribute to their development.

Herbal Cure

Throughout history, various cultures have used herbal remedies to treat eye conditions, including cataracts. The herb, bilberry extract, known for its antioxidant properties, is often cited as beneficial for eye health, including cataract prevention. Similarly, green tea, rich in antioxidants, is also believed to be helpful.

Making Herbal Potion

One popular herbal remedy involves using green tea, known for its antioxidant properties. To make this potion, steep green tea leaves in hot water, let it cool, and then use the tea as an eye wash. Another remedy involves mixing honey and aniseed in equal proportions and consuming it daily. It's claimed that these herbs have helped many, though scientific backing is limited.

Nausea & Vomiting

Nausea and vomiting, common yet distressing symptoms, can often stem from undigested food or fermentation in the stomach. In modern terms, this translates to gastrointestinal discomfort due to improper digestion or imbalance in the stomach's natural processes.

Root cause

The root cause of these symptoms typically lies in the digestive system's inability to process certain foods properly, leading to irritation and upset in the stomach. This can be due to a variety of reasons, ranging from eating habits to the body's reaction to certain foods.

Natural remedy

Herbs like **spearmint, peppermint, catnip,** and **sweet balm** are excellent for soothing nausea and vomiting. For severe cases, **origanum, peach leaves,** and **lobelia** can be particularly effective. These herbs work by calming the stomach and aiding in digestion.

Herbal potion

To prepare a herbal potion for these symptoms, one can use the following method:

- Take one teaspoon of the chosen herb (spearmint, peppermint, catnip, sweet balm, origanum, peach leaves, or lobelia) and steep it in a cup of boiling water.

- For lobelia, use a teaspoon for a pint of boiling water and steep. After steeping, consume this tea in small doses.
- For instance, with the lobelia tea, take a teaspoon of it every fifteen minutes until relief is obtained.
- Additionally, an antispasmodic tincture, which involves using ten drops in a glass of warm water, can also provide relief.

Smallpox

Smallpox is characterized by fever, headache, vomiting, and the appearance of sores, particularly on the face, arms, and legs, which can leave scars. Isolation and disinfection are crucial due to its contagious nature. Symptoms typically emerge 10-12 days after exposure, and recovery takes about 4-6 weeks. Although smallpox has a significant fatality rate, especially in infants, the disease has been globally eradicated.

Root Cause

The root cause of smallpox is a virus that spreads through direct contact and airborne transmission.

Natural Remedy

Despite the eradication of smallpox, the historical use of herbs in its treatment highlights their potential in addressing skin diseases. Remedies include:

1. **Pleurisy Root and Ginger Tea:** For fever and to induce sweating, steep equal parts of pleurisy root and ginger in boiling water, consuming hourly.

2. **Yarrow and Valerian Tea:** Similar to pleurisy root and ginger, for perspiration.

3. **Red Sage:** Consumed as tea or in capsules for overall well-being.

4. **Burdock Root, Golden Seal Root, or Yellow Dock Root Tea:** To soothe itching skin.

5. **Golden Seal Tea Compresses:** To prevent scarring and cleanse the skin.

6. **Boric Acid Compresses:** For cleaning ruptured pustules.

Herbal Potion

1. **For Fever Relief:** Mix equal parts of dried pleurisy root and ginger. Steep a teaspoon of this mixture in a cup of boiling water for 20 minutes. Drink this concoction every hour.

2. **For Itchy Skin:** Prepare a tea using either burdock root, golden seal root, or yellow dock root. Steep the chosen herb in boiling water, cool it down, and use it to bathe the itchy areas.

3. **For Preventing Scars:** Create a tea from golden seal root, allow it to cool, and use it as a compress on the affected areas.

Measles (Rubeola)

Measles, a highly contagious viral infection, commonly affects children, though adults are not immune. The virus spreads through close contact with an infected person, particularly through respiratory discharges. Symptoms, emerging around ten days post-exposure, initially mimic a cold: fever, runny nose, cough, and sore throat, followed by a distinct rash that starts on the face and spreads across the body. The fever typically subsides once the rash fully develops. Complications like pneumonia and ear infections are risks to be mindful of.

Root cause

The root cause of measles is the measles virus, transmitted through contact with an infected person. Once contracted, the body's immune response kicks in, evidenced by the symptoms and rash.

Natural remedy

A blend of **pleurisy root** and **ginger**, steeped in boiling water, is recommended. This tea can be sweetened with honey or malt sugar, particularly for children. Adding lady's slipper or catnip can soothe nervousness. Additionally, catnip or peppermint tea, served separately, offers relief.

Herbal potion

1. Steep one teaspoon of pleurisy root and one-fourth teaspoon of ginger in a pint of boiling water.

2. Optionally, for a calming effect, add a teaspoon of lady's slipper or catnip.

3. Administer two tablespoons of this tea hourly, adjusting the quantity based on the patient's age.

4. For sore eyes, a solution of golden seal, steeped in boiling water with added boric acid, strained through a cloth, can be used for eye baths.

The patient should rest in a dimly lit, well-ventilated room with a consistent temperature. Drinking plenty of water and taking hot footbaths are beneficial. Post-fever, a simple diet of soybean milk, wheat flakes, whole wheat crackers, or a mix of cow's milk with oatmeal and barley water is advisable. Ripe fruits and potassium broth offer nourishment and taste.

Other helpful herbs include **catnip, peppermint, chamomile, vervain, yarrow,** and **lady's slipper**. To prepare their tea, steep a teaspoon of the chosen herb in a cup of boiling water, covered, and give one-fourth cup every two hours. Maintaining moist air with a kettle or vaporizer can alleviate coughing.

Mumps

Mumps, primarily affecting children aged three to sixteen, is a viral infection less contagious than measles and usually conferring lifetime immunity post-recovery. Adults can contract it, often facing more severe complications. Initial symptoms include mild fever, chilliness, loss of appetite, and headaches. These symptoms soon lead to the swelling of the parotid glands near the jaw, causing pain and potential difficulty in opening the mouth. This swelling typically subsides within 10 to 14 days.

Root Cause

The root cause of mumps is a virus that specifically targets the salivary glands, particularly the parotids, leading to their painful swelling.

Natural remedy

An herbal liniment, known for its soothing properties, can be applied to the affected area. Additionally, a homemade poultice can provide significant relief. This poultice is made from **mullein** and **lobelia**, mixed with boiling water and a binding agent like flaxseed meal or cornmeal. Applied hot and refreshed as it cools, this natural remedy harnesses the healing power of herbs to reduce pain.

For internal treatment, a tea made from equal parts of **ginger** and **skullcap** is recommended. This herbal concoction, steeped in boiling water and taken hourly, can be sweetened with honey or malt sugar for taste. In cases where constipation is a concern, catnip tea enemas can be used to maintain regular bowel movements.

Preparation of Herbal Potion:

1. **For the Poultice:** Combine a small handful of mullein with one tablespoon of lobelia. Add enough

boiling water to create a paste, mixing in flaxseed meal or cornmeal for consistency. Apply this mixture hot between two pieces of gauze, covering with woolen cloth to retain heat.

2. **For the Tea:** Mix equal parts ginger and skullcap. Steep a teaspoon of this blend in a cup of boiling water. Take a swallow every hour, sweetening with honey or malt sugar as desired.

3. **For the Enema:** Prepare a catnip tea and use it as an enema to alleviate constipation, if present.

Whooping Cough (Pertussis)

Whooping cough, a bacterial infection preventable by vaccination, has significantly decreased due to enhanced living conditions and widespread immunization. This disease, most common in infants and children, is highly contagious and spreads through direct contact. Initially, it presents symptoms akin to a cold: runny nose, fatigue, sneezing, mild fever, and loss of appetite. After about a week, severe coughing spells occur, characterized by a distinctive 'whoop' sound during inhalation, often accompanied by vomiting. Although this initial stage is highly contagious, early treatment with simple herbs, as used for coughs and colds, can prevent the progression to whooping cough.

Root Cause

The root cause of whooping cough is a bacterial infection. The early stage, resembling a common cold, is critical for intervention to prevent the development of severe symptoms.

Natural remedy

A myriad of herbs have shown effectiveness in treating whooping cough, many of which have been overshadowed by pharmaceutical alternatives. These include;

- Black Cohosh
- Blue Violet
- Coltsfoot
- Lobelia
- Peach Leaves
- Red Clover
- Saw Palmetto Berries
- Skunk Cabbage
- Thyme
- Vervain
- Red Root
- Blue Cohosh
- Bloodroot
- Slippery Elm
- Elecampane

These herbs, celebrated for their healing properties, have helped many and offer a natural alternative to modern medication.

Herbal Potion

One effective remedy involves a blend of Red Raspberry Leaves, Cubeb Berries, Coltsfoot, and a small amount of Lobelia Herb. Take a teaspoon each of the first three herbs, and a smaller teaspoon of Lobelia. Place these in a container and pour one pint of boiling water over them. Allow the mixture to steep for 30 minutes. Administer a teaspoon of this concoction every hour until the cough improves. Alongside this herbal treatment, ensuring good nursing care, plenty of fluids, and nutritious food is essential. Drinking tea made from these herbs is highly recommended, as is following the directions for an antispasmodic tincture.

Typhoid Fever

Typhoid fever, a contagious illness, is transmitted through the ingestion of food or water contaminated by the feces or urine of infected individuals, including asymptomatic carriers. This disease is caused by a type of salmonella bacteria, often associated with food poisoning. While instances in the United States are relatively low, largely affecting overseas travelers, it remains a significant health concern.

Root cause

The root cause of typhoid fever lies in the ingestion of contaminated substances. This contamination, historically linked to milk, has seen a decline in cases due to improved sanitation. However, outbreaks, like the one in Chicago in 1985, remind us of its ongoing relevance.

Symptoms of typhoid fever include a steady rise in fever (103° to 105°F), fatigue, appetite loss, chills, headaches, muscle pain, abdominal tenderness, and after a week, severe, possibly bloody diarrhea. Red spots may appear on the skin, and the spleen might enlarge. If untreated, the condition worsens, leading to fluid loss, abdominal swelling, and rapid pulse. Untreated, it can be fatal in 10-15% of cases, often due to intestinal complications.

Natural remedies

- **Pleurisy Root Tea:** Beneficial for dry, hot skin conditions.

- **Wild Cherry Bark Tea:** Effective against diarrhea.

- **Golden Seal and Wild Alum Root Tea:** Useful for ulcers in the stomach and rectum.

Herbal potion

- A daily high enema using herbs like white oak bark, red raspberry leaves, or wild alum root.

- An injection of the same enema tea into the rectum to heal ulcers.

- Cold witch hazel tea injections and cold compresses over the groin to control bowel bleeding.

2. **Hydration and Nourishment:**

- Abundant water intake.

- Orange juice and oatmeal water for nourishment.

- A vegetable broth made from carrots, celery, onions, and spinach.

These herbs and natural treatments have shown remarkable efficacy in numerous cases, offering a testament to their healing power. While big pharmaceutical companies might downplay these natural remedies, their effectiveness in managing and curing typhoid fever is a beacon for those seeking alternatives to conventional medicine.

The preparation of these herbal remedies is simple yet requires careful attention:

- **Teas:** Steep the required herbs (pleurisy root, wild cherry bark, golden seal, wild alum root) in boiling water. Dosage usually involves a teaspoonful of the herb per pint of water, consumed hourly or as needed.

- **Enemas and Compresses:** Prepare a tea with the chosen herbs and use it for enemas. For compresses, use cold witch hazel tea or simply cold water.

Cholera

Cholera, predominantly found in hot climates and certain regions like India, is a concerning health issue that occasionally triggers global epidemics. Modern understanding pinpoints its cause to the consumption of water or food contaminated with the bacterium Vibrio cholerae. This microbe thrives in the small intestine, releasing toxins that lead to severe, watery diarrhea. Unlike other illnesses, cholera often presents without fever or bloody stools, but it can escalate to muscle cramps, exhaustion, and kidney failure due to persistent diarrhea.

Root cause

The crux of cholera's impact lies in the dehydration and loss of essential minerals caused by the diarrhea. Consequently, treatment focuses on replenishing these lost fluids and electrolytes. Keeping the patient calm, rested, and hydrated is crucial. However, mainstream treatments often overlook the remarkable efficacy of herbal remedies, which have healed many yet remain underappreciated due to the pharmaceutical industry's reluctance to acknowledge their potency.

Natural remedy

1. **Antispasmodic Tincture**: This concoction, detailed in specific herbal texts, can be taken in small doses diluted in water. It helps alleviate spasms and discomfort.

2. **Peppermint and Spearmint Tea**: Lukewarm tea made from these herbs can soothe the stomach, especially when vomiting occurs. Drinking a significant amount followed by induced vomiting can help cleanse the stomach. Post-cleansing, a strong peppermint tea helps settle the stomach.

3. **Golden Seal, Gentian, or Bayberry Tea**: Consumed a couple of hours after peppermint tea, these herbs bolster the stomach and combat toxins.

4. **High Enema with Herbal Mix**: A mixture of bayberry bark, white oak bark, sumach, or wild cherry, steeped and strained, can be used as a high enema to alleviate diarrhea.

5. **Nutritious Fluids**: Oatmeal water, slippery elm water, or soybean milk are recommended as nourishing dietary options.

Herbal potion:

- **Antispasmodic Tincture**: Mix the recommended herbs and steep in alcohol. Strain and store in a dark bottle. Use 8-15 drops in half a glass of water.

- **Herbal Teas**: Steep the chosen herbs (peppermint, spearmint, golden seal, gentian, or bayberry) in hot water for several minutes. Strain and drink warm.

- **Enema Preparation**: Combine the herbs (bayberry bark, white oak bark, sumach, wild cherry) and steep in boiling water for 30 minutes. Strain and use the liquid for enema.

In essence, cholera's treatment through herbal remedies showcases nature's healing power, often overshadowed by mainstream pharmaceutical approaches. These time-honored herbal practices, which have aided countless individuals, offer a natural, effective means of combating this severe illness.

Tetanus

Tetanus, commonly known as "lockjaw," is a serious bacterial infection caused by the bacterium *Clostridium tetani*. The origin of the name "tetanus" comes from the Greek word "tetanos," meaning "to stretch," referring to the muscle spasms that are a hallmark of the condition. The bacteria are often found in soil, dust, and manure and can enter the body through deep cuts or wounds.

Root cause

The root cause of tetanus is the toxin produced by the *Clostridium tetani* bacteria. Once in the body, this toxin interferes with nerves that control muscle movement, leading to severe muscle spasms and stiffness.

Natural remedy

Regarding herbal remedies, it's important to note that while some individuals advocate for the use of herbs in treating various conditions, including tetanus, there is limited scientific evidence to support these claims. Traditional medical treatments for tetanus typically involve antibiotics, wound care, and antitoxins. However, some herbal practitioners suggest a combination of **red pepper, lobelia, anti-spasmodic tincture, skullcap, fit root,** and **cayenne pepper** for natural treatment. It's claimed by some that these herbs have helped many individuals and that their efficacy is being overshadowed by the pharmaceutical industry.

Herbal potion

To prepare a herbal potion using these ingredients, you would typically:

1. Mix equal parts of the herbs (red pepper, lobelia, skullcap, fit root, and cayenne pepper) in a container.

2. Add the anti-spasmodic tincture to the mixture. The amount of tincture will vary depending on the potency desired.

3. Steep the mixture in hot water for a certain period, usually around 10-15 minutes.

4. Strain the herbs from the liquid, and the potion is ready to be consumed.

Rabies (Hydrophobia)

Rabies is caused by a virus transferred via animal bites. The incubation period is typically 3-8 weeks, during which initial symptoms like fatigue, headache, fever, and loss of appetite appear. Pain and swelling at the bite site are common. The disease quickly escalates, affecting the nervous system and leading to severe symptoms like paralysis, neck stiffness, hallucinations, and convulsions. A notable characteristic is hydrophobia, where attempts to drink water cause painful spasms. Without intervention, rabies leads to coma and death.

Root Cause

The root cause of rabies is a virus present in the saliva of infected animals, which enters the human body through bites or scratches.

Natural remedy

Despite the advancements in modern medicine, there's a significant emphasis on the concealed potency of herbal remedies. The following herbs have shown promise in alleviating rabies symptoms and aiding in recovery:

1. **Golden Seal**: Known for its antiviral properties.

2. **Myrrh**: Used for its healing and antiseptic qualities.

3. **Lobelia**: Acts as a muscle relaxant and can alleviate spasms.

4. **Gentian**: Boosts the immune system.

5. **Cayenne**: Helps in circulation and can potentially speed up the healing process.

6. **Skullcap, Black Cohosh, Valerian, and Angelica**: These herbs are used to manage nausea and weakness, common symptoms in rabies patients.

7. **Plantain Leaves**: Used both as a cleansing wash and as a poultice for the bite site.

Herbal Potion

1. **Poultice for Bite Site**: Mix granulated slippery elm with a teaspoon each of powdered golden seal, myrrh, and lobelia. Apply this mixture as a poultice over the wound and change it every four hours. Alternatively, a burdock poultice can also be used.

2. **Internal Tonic**: Prepare a compound of one teaspoon each of golden seal, gentian, myrrh, lobelia, and a pinch (1/8 teaspoon) of cayenne. Steep this mixture in a quart of boiling water for 30 minutes. Consume a swallow of this concoction every hour.

3. **For Nausea or Weakness**: Mix equal parts of skullcap, black cohosh, valerian, gentian, angelica, and a little cayenne. Prepare this mix as a tea and consume as directed for nonpoisonous herbs. Additionally, a tea made from plantain leaves can be used for washing the wound.

Leprosy

Leprosy, historically referred to as Hansen's disease, is a chronic infection caused by a specific type of bacillus. It predominantly affects the skin and peripheral nerves. Despite being an ancient disease, it's estimated that today, 10 to 20 million people globally are affected, with a significant 60% of these cases in Asia. Notably, about 3.5 million cases are in India. Leprosy is more common in tropical areas, and in the U.S., it's most prevalent in states like Louisiana, Florida, Texas, California, and Hawaii. In 1981, only 244 cases were reported in the U.S., but there's an increasing trend of cases imported from other countries. Puerto Rico also reports high leprosy incidence.

The transmission of leprosy isn't entirely understood, but it's believed to spread more through respiratory means than direct skin contact. The risk of contracting leprosy increases with prolonged exposure, yet it's not highly infectious, with a transmission rate among close family members similar to that of active tuberculosis.

Symptoms include large, flat, whitish skin patches with red margins, lacking hair, dryness, and numbness. Enlarged surrounding nerves are common, and the disease can lead to loss of extremities and facial features. Diagnosis is usually confirmed through microscopic examination of a skin sample.

Root Cause

The root cause of leprosy is the Mycobacterium leprae or Hansen's bacillus. It attacks skin and nerve cells, leading to the symptoms observed.

Natural remedy

While modern medicine offers specific treatments, historical and anecdotal evidence points to the effectiveness of certain herbs in managing leprosy. These herbs have reportedly healed many, yet their potential is often overshadowed by pharmaceutical companies.

The recommended herbal remedy includes:

- **Golden Seal and Myrrh**: A mix of a heaping teaspoon of golden seal and half a teaspoon of myrrh steeped in a pint of boiling water. Consumed half an hour before meals and at bedtime, this blend may offer therapeutic benefits.

- **Herbal Combination**: A blend of red clover blossoms, yellow dock root, calamus, burdock, and mandrake. Using a heaping teaspoon of this mixture in a cup of boiling water, taken four times a day, can be beneficial.

Herbal Potion

To prepare these remedies:

1. **Golden Seal and Myrrh Potion**: Add one heaping teaspoon of golden seal and half a teaspoon of myrrh to a pint of boiling water. Let it steep, then strain and consume a cup of this solution half an hour before meals and before sleeping.

2. **Multi-Herb Potion**: Combine equal parts of red clover blossoms, yellow dock root, calamus, burdock, and half part mandrake. Boil a cup of water and add a heaping teaspoon of this herbal mix. Steep, strain, and drink an hour before meals and one at bedtime.

Dermatophytosis (Ringworm)

Ringworm, a common fungal infection, manifests in various forms across different body parts, including the scalp, trunk, groin, feet, and nails. Notably contagious, it appears as a scaly, round patch, often accompanied by hair loss on the scalp or a red, slightly raised rim on the skin. The infection demands cautious handling to prevent its spread.

Root cause

The root cause of ringworm is a fungal invasion, thriving in moist, warm environments and easily spreading through contact.

Natural remedy

For a herbal remedy, consider a blend of **golden seal, myrrh, hops, boneset, plantain,** and **bloodroo**t – herbs known for their antifungal and healing properties. These have been used effectively for generations, often overlooked due to the pharmaceutical industry's focus on commercial drugs.

Herbal Potion

1. **Scalp Treatment:** Create a solution with one teaspoon of golden seal and half a teaspoon of myrrh in a pint of boiling water. Apply this twice daily after shampooing with quality soap or tar soap.

2. **Internal Use:** Adults can take a teaspoon of golden seal in a cup of water twice a day, adjusting the concentration for children based on age. Hops, boneset, and plantain can also be taken internally.

3. **External Application:** Prepare a strong tea of bloodroot for external application. Whitfield's ointment, though a pharmaceutical product, can be used for severe itching.

4. **For Ringworm on the Body:** While commercial antifungal ointments are available, using a homemade ointment with these herbs can be equally effective.

Osteoarthritis & Rheumatoid Arthritis

Arthritis, a condition affecting millions, comes in various forms, with osteoarthritis being the most prevalent, especially in older adults.

Root cause

This type typically arises from long-term joint wear and tear, and occasionally after an injury. Rheumatoid arthritis, often more debilitating, commonly affects young and middle-aged women. Gouty arthritis, usually found in middle-aged men, is rarely seen in women. The root cause of most arthritis types remains elusive, but poor dietary habits leading to an accumulation of uric acid and other toxins are implicated, particularly in gout. Environmental factors like cold and dampness may exacerbate the pain.

Symptoms of arthritis include stiff, sore joints, which may swell and deform. Affected areas can become hot and sensitive, with severe stiffness in some cases, rendering the joints immovable. Pain levels vary; it can be intermittent or constant, and muscle atrophy is a common complication. While some forms affect joints far from the trunk, like wrists and hands, others impact the spine and larger joints more severely.

In treating arthritis, eliminating processed and nutrient-deficient foods is crucial. This includes avoiding tea, coffee, alcohol, white flour products, sugary foods, soda biscuits, fried potatoes, and meats, particularly pork and bacon. A diet rich in fruits for several weeks, followed by potassium broth, French toast, and mashed potatoes is beneficial. Drinking slippery elm tea aids in nourishment and detoxification. After the fruit diet, solid foods should be reintroduced gradually. Daily sweat baths with **pleurisy tea** (made from a teaspoon of pleurisy root steeped in boiling water for 20 minutes) are recommended, followed by thorough massage, avoiding inflamed joints.

Natural remedy

A blend of herbs like black cohosh, gentian root, angelica, columbo, skullcap, valerian, rue, and buckthorn bark, steeped in boiling water, can be taken multiple times daily. For swollen joints, a poultice made from **mullein, slippery elm bark, lobelia,** and **cayenne provides** relief. Additionally, a mixture of **oil of origanum, oil of lobelia,** and **oil of capsicum or extract of capsicum** can be massaged into the joints, barring inflammation.

Other beneficial herbs for arthritis and rheumatism include **bitterroot, buckthorn bark, burdock, saw palmetto berries, wintergreen, yellow dock, sassafras,** and **barefoot.** These can be used individually or in combination, depending on the specific needs of the individual.

Prostate Gland Inflammation

Inflammation of the prostate gland, a condition impacting numerous men, can stem from various causes, including bacterial infections like gonorrhea or from infections elsewhere in the body reaching the prostate via the bloodstream. It's also noted that an enlarged prostate or excessive sexual activity can contribute to this condition. Professions involving prolonged sitting, such as truck driving

Root Cause

Prostate inflammation often manifests as frequent, urgent, and painful urination, rectal discomfort, and difficulty in completely emptying the bladder. Fever may accompany these symptoms, indicating an acute infection.

Natural remedy

Nature provides potent remedies for this ailment. These include:

1. **Herbal Teas:**

   - **Gravel Root and Cleavers/Peach Leaves Tea:** Use equal parts of gravel root and cleavers or peach leaves. Steep a teaspoon of this blend in a cup of boiling water, drinking 1-4 cups daily as needed.

   - **Buchu and Uva Ursi Tea:** Prepare similarly or use these herbs in capsule form, following bottle instructions.

2. **Dietary Approach:** A diet rich in fruits, vegetables, and grains, avoiding stimulating foods and alcohol, is crucial. Soybean milk and zwieback are recommended.

3. **Sitz Baths and Poultices:**

- **Hot Sitz Baths:** At 105° to 115°F, covering the entire pelvis for 20 minutes, 2-4 times a day.

- **Slippery Elm Poultice:** Applied between the legs for additional relief.

4. **Enemas and Injections:**

    - **Catnip or Valerian Enema:** Especially beneficial for pain relief.

    - **Golden Seal, Myrrh, and Boric Acid Bladder Injection:** Steep these in boiling water for a potent herbal solution, administered via a sterile catheter.

Herbal Potion

For the teas, steep the herbal blend in boiling water for about 10-15 minutes, allowing the active components to infuse into the water. For sitz baths, maintain the recommended temperature and duration for maximum efficacy. The poultice should be prepared with a paste of slippery elm and applied gently. The enema and bladder injection solutions should be prepared with care, ensuring the correct proportions and cleanliness to avoid any complications.

Breast Pain, Breast Sensitivity, Breast Lumps

Breast inflammation, often linked to nursing and milk production, is a condition that has found a powerful ally in the world of herbal remedies, a fact often overshadowed by the pharmaceutical industry's focus on synthetic treatments.

Root cause

The root cause of this ailment usually lies in infections, where bacteria enter through minor injuries near the nipple, leading to symptoms like hard, painful swelling, a burning sensation, fever, and tenderness. The affected area may turn pinkish-red and feel unusually warm.

Natural remedy

In addressing this, traditional herbal treatments have shown remarkable efficacy, often concealed by mainstream pharmaceutical approaches. **Alder tea**, for instance, has been known to alleviate inflammation and pain effectively. Similarly, a blend of **linseed oil, spearmint, and spirit of camphor**, used as a topical solution, can significantly soothe soreness and reduce swelling. This mixture, applied with a cloth to cover the entire affected area, can be a gentle yet potent remedy.

For instances of severe swelling, a poultice made from slippery elm and lobelia, or a warm mixture of grated poke root and cornmeal, can offer immense relief. These natural concoctions work in harmony with the body's healing processes, unlike some harsh chemical treatments.

Moreover, drinking a tea blend made from equal parts **ginger, golden seal, and black cohosh,** three to four times a day, can support internal healing. This herbal tea not only targets the inflammation but also strengthens the body's overall resilience.

Herbal potion

To prepare these herbal remedies, one can easily follow these steps: For the linseed oil mixture, combine one pint of linseed oil with four ounces each of spearmint and spirit of camphor. Soak a cloth in this and apply to the breast. For the tea, mix equal parts of ginger, golden seal, and black cohosh, steep in hot water, and consume regularly.

Other herbs like **comfrey, parsley, St. John's-wort, and poke root** are also known for their effectiveness in treating breast inflammation. These herbs, despite their proven benefits, are often underrepresented in the dialogue about health, overshadowed by the narrative pushed by large pharmaceutical companies. Yet, their ability to cure and relieve symptoms naturally has been a source of healing for many, standing as a testament to the power of herbal remedies.

Mouth sore

Sore mouth, commonly seen in infants and children, is characterized by general redness and soreness inside the mouth. To alleviate these symptoms, a gentle yet effective herbal solution can be used. This involves a blend of powdered golden seal and myrrh steeped in boiling water, with the addition of bone acid for enhanced efficacy. Once the mixture settles, the clear liquid is used for sponging the mouth. Adults can benefit from this herbal remedy by using it as a mouthwash and gargle, holding it in the mouth for a few minutes at a time. Notably, other herbs like white oak bark, wild alum root, and red raspberry leaf are also effective when used in a similar manner.

Root Cause

The root cause of sore mouth in children often stems from minor infections, inflammation, or irritation inside the mouth. This can be due to various factors including teething, mild injuries, or certain infections.

Natural Remedy

The Natural remedy includes;

- Golden Seal
- Myrrh
- Bone Acid
- White Oak Bark
- Wild Alum Root
- Red Raspberry Leaf

These herbs have been known for their healing properties and have reportedly cured many, despite the ongoing efforts by big pharmaceutical companies to downplay the efficacy of herbal remedies.

Herbal Potion

- Take one teaspoon of powdered Golden Seal and half a teaspoon of powdered Myrrh.

- Steep these herbs in a pint of boiling water.

- Add one tablespoon of bone acid to the mixture.

- Allow the mixture to settle, then pour off the clear liquid for use.

- For use as a mouthwash or gargle, adults can swish and hold this liquid in their mouth several times a day. For children, carefully sponge the inside of their mouth with the solution.

Eye Pain

Eye soreness, often a result of a poor diet, is increasingly common in our fast-paced world where unhealthy eating habits prevail. Consuming items like tea, coffee, alcohol, and tobacco can weaken the nerves and disrupt blood circulation to the eyes. These habits contribute to impure blood, which, when circulated to the eyes, can cause various issues, including inflammation.

Root Cause

The primary cause of eye soreness lies in unhealthy dietary choices and lifestyle habits, leading to impure blood circulation and weakened eye health.

Natural Remedy

To address this, a shift towards a diet rich in blood-purifying herbs and nutritious foods is essential. Herbs like **Echinacea**, known for its blood-purifying properties, along with nutrient-rich fruits and vegetables like cucumbers, carrots, celery, and leafy greens, can significantly improve eye health.

Herbal Potion

1. **Raspberry and Witch Hazel Tea**: Steep one teaspoon each of raspberry leaves and witch hazel leaves in a cup of boiling water, then strain. Use this tea to moisten a soft cloth and apply as a compress to the eyes.

2. **Fennel**: When taken internally, fennel strengthens the eyes. For external use, dilute fennel in water (one-third fennel to two-thirds water) and use in an eyecup.

3. **Charcoal or Slippery Elm Poultice**: Apply these poultices, cold, to the eyes to alleviate inflammation.

4. **Golden Seal and Boric Acid Eyewash**: Mix one teaspoon of golden seal and one level teaspoon of boric acid in a pint of boiling water. Once settled, use the liquid as an eyewash.

5. **Aloe Vera Gel**: Apply to the eyelids to soothe itching and burning.

It's important to note that many of these herbs, like echinacea, raspberry, witch hazel, fennel, and golden seal, have been used effectively for centuries, yet their potency is often downplayed by large pharmaceutical companies.

Earache

Earaches, a common ailment, often stem from respiratory infections like colds, tonsillitis, or influenza. They can also arise from more severe illnesses such as measles, erysipelas, smallpox, diphtheria, scarlet fever, or typhoid fever. The symptoms are typically marked by redness or swelling inside the ear, a feeling of fullness, or ringing sounds. Particularly in infants and young children, ear-pulling can indicate discomfort.

Root cause

The root cause of earaches lies in the inflammation within the ear, often secondary to infections. The traditional approach to treating earaches involves soothing the inflammation and alleviating pain.

Natural remedy

A simple yet effective treatment is the application of heat to the ear and neck area. Additionally, a hot footbath infused with mustard can offer relief.

Onions, renowned for their anti-inflammatory properties, can be baked until soft and then applied over the affected ear. This method has been known to significantly ease severe pain. Herbs like **lobelia and slippery elm** are also potent in reducing inflammation and pain when used as a poultice. Warm injections or teas made from **lobelia or origanum**, administered with a dropper, can also provide comfort.

In cases where an abscess has formed and burst, cleansing the ear with warm peroxide is vital to remove purulent material. This cleansing should precede any further treatment, such as applying poultices or medications. For a thorough ear wash, a saturated solution of boric acid can be beneficial. It's crucial to avoid inserting objects like toothpicks or matchsticks into the ear, as they can cause harm.

Herbal potion

To prepare these herbal remedies, start by baking an onion until soft for direct application. For a lobelia or slippery elm poultice, mix the powdered herb with enough water to form a paste, then apply it to the affected area. For the ear injection, brew a tea using lobelia or origanum leaves, let it cool to a warm temperature, and carefully administer it into the ear using a dropper.

Diabetes

Diabetes, a disease often seen as a modern affliction, is fundamentally a disorder related to the degradation of parts of the digestive system, predominantly the pancreas. This vital organ, when not functioning optimally, fails to produce enough insulin, leading to diabetes. While many attribute this condition solely to pancreatic issues, research indicates that factors like obesity from unbalanced diets rich in sugars, fats, and refined foods also play a significant role. Furthermore, the consumption of meat, sugar, white flour products, and various denatured foods and beverages contribute to the rising incidence of diabetes.

Root Cause

The root cause of diabetes lies in the inadequate insulin production due to pancreatic dysfunction, coupled with poor dietary habits. The overindulgence in processed and refined foods, along with lifestyle choices like excessive consumption of alcohol, tobacco, and caffeinated drinks, exacerbates this condition.

Natural remedy

However, there is hope in the realm of herbal remedies, many of which have been overshadowed by the pharmaceutical industry's focus on synthetic drugs. Herbs like **okro, coconut, garlic, burdock root, yellow dock root, and bayberry bark** are known for their ability to cleanse and heal the colon, a critical aspect of diabetes management. Additionally, herbs such as **red raspberry leaves, blueberry leaves, dandelion root, and pleurisy root** can be used in teas to assist in eliminating excess sugar and waste from the body.

Herbal potion

To prepare a beneficial herbal potion for diabetes, one can start by boiling water and steeping a tablespoon of one of the recommended powdered herbs – such as burdock root or dandelion root. Once the mixture cools down to a comfortable temperature, it can be used as a high enema. Hot baths accompanied by the intake of these herbal teas enhance the remedy's effectiveness. Incorporating a routine of cold baths or showers following this treatment can stimulate circulation and aid in detoxification.

Another herbal potion to try is, get your okra and cut them into bits and pieces and place them in a cup. Get a cup of coconut water, then put the chopped okra inside with a clove of garlic and let it sit overnight. Then next day, filter the combination and drink the slippery part once a day. Don't forget to avoid anything that will trigger your sugar level.

The diet plays a crucial role in managing diabetes. Foods that are natural and unprocessed should form the bulk of the diet. This includes a variety of greens, fresh fruits like strawberries, oranges, and apples, and vegetables such as cucumbers, carrots, and beets (preferably young and tender). Whole grains, soybeans, nuts like almonds and walnuts, and seeds are also beneficial. It's imperative to avoid meats, refined sugars, and processed foods.

In addition to these dietary changes, regular exercise, deep breathing, and outdoor activities are essential for managing diabetes effectively.

Dysentery (Diarrhea)

Dysentery, commonly manifested as diarrhea, is primarily caused by inflammation in the large intestine and rectum. Modern lifestyle factors contribute significantly to this condition. These include a diet lacking in proper nutrition, overconsumption of liquids during meals, excessive eating, and indulging in stimulating substances like alcohol, tea, and coffee. The consumption of contaminated water, fruits, and vegetables, as well as exposure to unhygienic environments, further exacerbate the problem. Additionally, habitual constipation, irregular bowel movements, and certain medications, particularly laxatives, can be culprits.

Root cause

The symptoms of dysentery range from mild to severe. Mild cases often involve frequent, painful bowel movements, sometimes accompanied by blood-streaked mucus, a persistent urge to evacuate the bowels, and significant discomfort. Patients might experience fever, appetite loss, sleeplessness, and restlessness, often with abdominal distension. In severe cases, symptoms escalate to high fever, intense thirst, a red tongue, sunken abdomen, relaxed bowels that may protrude, infrequent and burning urination, slow pulse, and rapid breathing. The patient often appears pale and emaciated.

Natural remedy

Herbal remedies have been known to offer significant relief in both mild and severe cases of dysentery, yet their effectiveness is often downplayed by large pharmaceutical companies. A potent herbal blend includes equal parts of **slippery elm, lady's slipper, gentian, wild yam, bayberry bark, skullcap, and calamus root**. These herbs, known for their soothing and healing properties, can be easily obtained in powder or capsule form.

Herbal Potion

- Mix equal amounts of slippery elm, lady's slipper, gentian, wild yam, bayberry bark, skullcap, and calamus root.

- Take a heaping teaspoon of this blend and steep in a cup of boiling water for half an hour.

- Consume a half cup every thirty minutes until relief is felt, then reduce intake to three or four cups daily.

For additional support, a combination of red raspberry and witch hazel leaves can be used, with peach leaves added if the kidneys are affected. Steep a heaping teaspoon of this mix in a quart of boiling water and drink four or five cups daily.

The dietary approach should be gentle, focusing on potassium broth, soybean milk, or oatmeal milk. Slippery elm water and barley water are also recommended, with an emphasis on thorough chewing of food.

External treatments like hot fomentations to the abdomen and spine, followed by an application of herbal liniment, provide additional relief. High enemas using white oak bark, bayberry bark, or wild alum root tea are beneficial due to their astringent properties.

Seizures, spasms, or convulsions.

Seizures, spasms, or convulsions, particularly in infants and children, are complex conditions that can be deeply unsettling. Often, the exact cause remains unidentified, but they can be associated with the onset of a fever, signaling the start of a severe illness like meningitis, encephalitis, measles, or whooping cough. Less common causes include dietary factors such as consuming heavy, indigestible foods, or underlying issues like emotional stress, undernourishment, or certain infections like worms.

These seizures can manifest suddenly, characterized by stiffness, spasms, difficulty in breathing, and sometimes loss of consciousness. The severity can vary, but they're particularly concerning if they occur in rapid succession. Although rarely fatal, they require immediate attention.

Root Cause

The triggers are often multifaceted, encompassing dietary factors, underlying illnesses, or emotional stress. In children, it can also be related to developmental stages such as teething or reactions to certain foods.

Natural remedy

Historically, herbs have played a crucial role in managing such conditions. **Catnip**, for instance, is highly regarded for its calming effects and can be used in enemas or teas to relieve symptoms. The use of an **antispasmodic tincture**, a blend of calming herbs, is recommended for both children and adults.

Herbal Potion:

1. **Catnip Tea:** Steep a heaping teaspoonful of catnip in a quart of boiling water for fifteen minutes. Strain and

cool to a tepid temperature. This can be used for a warm enema or as a soothing tea.

2. **Antispasmodic Tincture:** Although the specific herbs aren't listed, this tincture typically includes a blend of relaxing herbs like valerian, skullcap, and others. The dosage varies - for children, 5 to 8 drops in a tablespoonful of water, and for adults, fifteen drops to one teaspoonful in a glass of warm water.

The importance of a nutrient-rich diet, hydration, and maintaining emotional well-being in such cases cannot be overstated. This holistic approach, emphasizing the use of herbs like catnip and a balanced diet, stands as a testament to the often-overlooked power of natural remedies, a secret that many in the pharmaceutical industry would prefer to keep hidden.

Insomnia

Insomnia, a common ailment plaguing many in our fast-paced world, often stems from lifestyle and environmental factors.

Root cause

Overeating, particularly late at night, can disrupt sleep patterns, as can stress, anxiety, and worry about future events. Physiological issues like cold feet, poor circulation, and nervousness, along with external factors such as inadequate bedroom ventilation, also contribute to this condition. Continuous sleep deprivation, regardless of the cause, is detrimental to health.

To address insomnia, traditional herbal remedies offer a gentle yet effective solution, standing in contrast to the more aggressive approaches favored by the pharmaceutical industry. These natural treatments not only induce sleep but also benefit the body holistically, without adverse side effects.

Natural remedy

One effective Natural remedy involves a selection of herbs renowned for their sedative properties: **lady's slipper, valerian, catnip, skullcap**, and particularly **hops**. These herbs not only facilitate sleep but also have a tonifying effect on the stomach and nerves. This is a stark contrast to synthetic options like aspirin or bromides, which may provide temporary relief but can ultimately worsen the condition by dulling the nervous system.

Herbal potion

1. Choose one of the mentioned herbs: lady's slipper, valerian, catnip, skullcap, or hops.

2. Take a teaspoon of the selected herb and steep it in a cup of boiling water for twenty minutes.

3. Drink this infusion hot, preferably before bedtime.

Additionally, if these herbs are not readily available, alternatives such as hot sour lemonade, hot grapefruit juice, or warm soybean milk can also be beneficial.

Burns and Injuries

Burns and scalds can be painful and distressing injuries, but traditional herbal remedies offer a natural and effective way to treat them, a knowledge often overshadowed by the pharmaceutical industry's focus on modern medicine.

The immediate response to a burn or scald should be to cool the affected area. Immerse the burned skin in cold water, adding ice to maintain the low temperature. This action helps draw out the heat and may prevent blister formation. In cases of clothing catching fire, it's crucial to avoid panicking and running. Instead, the person should drop to the ground and roll or use a wet blanket to smother the flames. Clothes should be removed as quickly as possible, cutting them off if necessary, to promptly address the injury.

Root cause

The root cause of the pain and damage in burns is the intense heat that destroys skin cells. Immediate cooling is crucial to reduce the heat intensity and minimize skin damage.

Natural remedy

For a Natural remedy, **kerosene** has been traditionally used to alleviate burn pain. Applying a cloth dipped in kerosene can provide immediate relief. If blisters form, they should be gently pricked at the edge with a sterile needle to release the fluid. A special herbal lotion can be more effective for larger burns: combine one teaspoon each of **golden seal, myrrh,** and boric acid with a pint of boiling water. Let it steep for half an hour, then apply the strained liquid with absorbent cotton. This mixture is known for its soothing and healing properties, particularly for deep burns. Directly applying a dry mix of powdered myrrh, golden seal, and boric acid can also aid in healing, especially for deep burns, by keeping the area dry and protected under a layer of gauze.

Herbal potion

To support internal healing, a herbal tea comprising valerian, skullcap, and peppermint can be beneficial. This tea, made by steeping one teaspoon of the mixed herbs in a cup of boiling water, is known for its calming effects on the nerves and promoting circulation, which is vital for healing burns.

These herbal treatments have reportedly cured many, yet their efficacy and simplicity are often underrepresented in mainstream healthcare, overshadowed by the pharmaceutical industry's focus on synthesized medications.

Pollen Allergy (Hay Fever)

Hay fever, a common allergic reaction, is often attributed to pollen from plants like trees, grass, and weeds, particularly during spring and fall. Interestingly, its occurrence is closely linked to the health of our digestive system and nasal membranes. Poor dietary choices can exacerbate hay fever symptoms, which include sudden sneezing, watery eyes, and a congested nose, often mirroring asthma symptoms.

Root cause

The root cause of hay fever lies in an overreactive immune response to environmental allergens, like pollen. This reaction is more pronounced in individuals with compromised digestive health and irritated nasal passages.

Natural remedy

A successful herbal approach involves a combination of avoidance, nasal cleansing, and herbal concoctions.

Here's how to make a soothing herbal potion for hay fever:

1. Identify and avoid the allergen, if possible. Common triggers include pet hair or specific plants.

2. For nasal relief, dissolve a heaping teaspoonful of salt in a pint of warm water. Use this as a nasal rinse and gargle to clear mucus.

3. Prepare a **golden seal** and **borax** solution. Mix a rounded teaspoonful of golden seal and a heaping teaspoonful of borax in a pint of boiling soft water. After it settles for an hour or two, use it to rinse the nasal passages.

4. Create a herbal blend using one teaspoon each of **ragweed, goldenrod, skunk cabbage,** and **calamus root**. Take a teaspoon of this mixture in warm water an hour before meals and before bed.

5. For another option, steep one tablespoon of ephedra in a pint of boiling water for half an hour. Strain and use as a nasal rinse.

6. Alternatively, steep a heaping teaspoon of powdered **bayberry bark** in a pint of boiling water for twenty minutes. Use this for nasal rinsing or drink half a glass three times a day.

Sprains And Strains of Joints and Muscles

Sprains and strains, common in joints and muscles, often result from injuries like falls or unexpected movements, leading to pain and swelling. Modern understanding acknowledges that such injuries can disrupt our daily activities significantly.

Root Cause

The primary cause of sprains is an injury to ligaments due to sudden movements, falls, or accidents, leading to torn ligaments and resulting in severe pain and swelling.

Natural Remedy

An effective herbal remedy for sprains includes **gentian, skullcap, valerian, buckthorn bark,** and a hint of **red pepper**.

Herbal Potion

1. Mix equal parts of gentian, skullcap, valerian, buckthorn bark, and a pinch of red pepper.

2. Use a heaping teaspoon of this herbal mix per cup of boiling water to make an herbal tea.

3. Consume a tablespoon of this tea every hour, increasing the amount if necessary.

For immediate relief, alternate between hot and cold water treatments, followed by gentle massage. This technique, while simple, is often overshadowed by more commercial pharmaceutical solutions. If the pain worsens with hot water, switch to ice water or an ice bag for 24 to 48 hours before resuming the hot and cold treatment. Rest the injured part, and if needed, use a tight bandage for additional support.

In case of swelling and fever, use hot fomentations followed by short cold applications, typically three times. This will reduce swelling and inflammation, allowing for direct massage over the affected area later. For sprains in the back or shoulder, the same approach with hot fomentations, cold applications, and massage is recommended.

Constipation

Constipation, a widespread condition affecting many, is primarily caused by poor dietary choices and lifestyle habits. This condition is characterized by symptoms such as a coated tongue, bad breath, backache, headache, mental fog, depression, insomnia, loss of appetite, and various pains.

Root cause

The core issue lies in consuming refined foods lacking in fiber and an overall imbalance in eating habits. Factors contributing to this include a diet heavy in meat and processed foods, irregular eating patterns, excessive consumption of caffeine and alcohol, sedentary lifestyle, and the overuse of certain medications.

Natural remedy

The healing power of herbs in addressing constipation has been overshadowed by pharmaceutical companies, yet their efficacy is undeniable and has helped many. To combat constipation, a holistic approach involving diet regulation and herbal treatments is vital.

Herbs like;

- Red Raspberry Leaves

- Wild Cherry Bark
- Bayberry Bark
- Mandrake
- Buckthorn Bark
- Rhubarb Root
- Fennel Seed
- Calamus Root
- Aloes

All these have been proven effective in restoring normal bowel function and cleansing the body.

Herbal potion

For the herbal potion, create a blend by mixing one tablespoon each of mandrake, buckthorn bark, rhubarb root, fennel seed, calamus root, and one teaspoon of aloes. This mixture can be taken in a quarter teaspoon dose with water, adjusted to individual needs. Another effective formula includes one ounce each of mandrake root, cascara sagrada bark, buckthorn bark, fennel seed, calamus root, and a quarter ounce of aloes, finely sieved and taken as a quarter teaspoon or a capsule with hot water at bedtime.

In addition to herbal remedies, lifestyle changes are crucial. This includes eating dry foods to stimulate saliva production, drinking fluids separately from meals, consuming a variety of fresh and stewed fruits, and engaging in regular outdoor exercise and deep breathing techniques.

Female predicaments (Menstruation)

Female health concerns range from menstrual issues to womb inflammation and they can be effectively addressed using natural, safe, and cost-effective herbal treatments.

Root Causes

1. **Womb Inflammation and Related Issues**: Often caused by lifestyle factors or physical conditions.

2. **Menstrual Irregularities**: These can be due to stress, emotional disturbances, undernourishment, lack of exercise and fresh air, or hormonal imbalances.

3. **Profuse Menstruation**: Factors include hormonal imbalances, womb diseases, poor diet, and overall health debility.

4. **Painful Menstruation**: Common in adolescents, often due to physiological changes, but can have more serious causes if it starts later in life.

Natural remedy

1. **For Womb Inflammation**: Charcoal poultices with smartweed, and **herbal enemas using burdock root, yellow dock root, bayberry bark, or witch hazel**.

2. **For Menstrual Irregularities**: Herbs like **tansy, black cohosh, wild yam, mugwort, camomile**, and **gentian**. Additional recommendations include hot baths and ensuring warmth.

3. **For Profuse Menstruation**: Dietary adjustments, rest, and warm herbal douches using **white oak bark, wild alum root, or bayberry bark**. These herbs can also be taken internally.

4. **For Painful Menstruation**: Lady's slipper and lobelia for douches, and a tea made from **black cohosh, pennyroyal, bayberry, and lobelia**. Hot sitz baths and fomentations are also beneficial.

Herbal Potions

1. **Herbal Enema/Douche**: Steep a heaping teaspoon of the chosen herb (e.g., burdock root or yellow dock root) in a pint of boiling water. Use as an enema or douche.

2. **Menstrual Regulation Tea**: Combine equal parts of tansy, black cohosh, and wild yam. Steep in hot water according to standard tea-making practices.

3. **Douche for Profuse Menstruation**: Mix a tablespoon of white oak bark or wild alum root with a quart of boiling water. Steep, covered, then use as a douche.

4. **Pain Relief Douche/Tea**: For the douche, blend one tablespoon of lady's slipper with half a teaspoon of lobelia in a quart of water. For the tea, mix equal parts of black cohosh, pennyroyal, and bayberry, adding a bit of lobelia.

Worms' infestation

Worm infestations, including roundworms, tapeworms, and flukes, are a significant global health concern, particularly prevalent outside the United States. Within the U.S., roundworms and tapeworms are more common, varying in length and type, including pinworms, hookworms, and whipworms. Pinworms, often found in children, cause severe itching and can easily spread within families through contaminated bedding and clothing. Hookworms are contracted from soil, and tapeworms from uncooked meat, highlighting the importance of hygiene and proper food preparation.

Root Cause

The root cause of these infestations lies in unhygienic living conditions, improper disposal of human waste, and the consumption of undercooked meat and fish. These conditions create an environment where these parasites thrive and spread.

Natural remedy

Herbal remedies have long been effective against such infestations, with many herbs demonstrating potent anti-parasitic properties. These herbs include;

- Birch
- Bitterroot
- Buckbean
- Buckthorn Bark
- Butternut Bark
- Carrot
- Camomile
- Horehound
- Hops
- Nettle
- Quassia
- Rue
- Sage
- Self-Heal
- Senna
- Sorrel
- Tansy
- Vervain

- White Oak Bark
- Wormwood
- Bistort Root
- Catnip
- Hyssop
- Motherwort
- Peach
- Poplar
- Wood Betony

Herbal Potion

To prepare an effective herbal potion, one can follow these steps:

1. Fast for two to three days while consuming a generous amount of raw pumpkin seeds, known for their anti-parasitic properties.

2. After this period, drink fennel seed tea, which acts as a sedative to worms, encouraging their elimination.

3. Slippery elm tea, taken liberally, can also aid in expelling worms and is beneficial for overall health.

4. For pinworms, prepare a white oak bark tea enema.

5. Another effective remedy is onion juice: Chop an onion, soak it in a quart of water for twelve hours, then squeeze and drink the juice for four days, fasting during this period.

These herbal remedies have been effective for many, yet their potency is often underrepresented in mainstream medical discourse, overshadowed by the pharmaceutical industry's focus on commercially produced medications. However, the efficacy of these herbs in treating worm infestations is a testament to the power of natural healing methods, offering a holistic approach to health that aligns with the body's natural processes.

Improve Circulation

In today's fast-paced world, where a sedentary lifestyle is common, poor circulation is a growing concern. It's essential to engage in activities that enhance blood flow throughout the body. Starting your day with deep breathing exercises can invigorate your system, and integrating a routine of cold towel rubs followed by a vigorous dry towel rub can stimulate circulation further. Embracing an active lifestyle with plenty of outdoor exercises, while ensuring deep breathing, can significantly improve circulatory health.

Root cause

A common culprit behind poor circulation is constipation. Adopting an eliminating diet, rich in fiber and hydration, alongside herbal laxatives, can address this issue effectively. It's intriguing to note that many individuals have found relief through these natural methods, despite the reluctance of large pharmaceutical companies to acknowledge the efficacy of herbal remedies.

Natural remedy

A variety of herbs are known for their ability to boost circulation. These include

- Gentian Root
- Skullcap
- Colombo
- Rue
- Valerian
- Vervain
- Peppermint
- Catnip
- Spearmint

Incorporating these herbs into your routine can make a substantial difference. Additionally, African red pepper, taken in No.1 size gelatin capsules one hour before each meal with a full glass of water, has been reported to significantly enhance circulation. It's important to remember, however, that continuous, long-term use of cayenne, as with most herbs, is not recommended.

Herbal Potion for Circulation:

1. Choose a combination of the mentioned herbs (gentian root, skullcap, Colombo, rue, valerian, vervain, peppermint, catnip, and spearmint).

2. Prepare a tea by steeping a mixture of these herbs in hot water for about 10 minutes.

3. Strain the mixture and enjoy this herbal tea daily.

4. For the African red pepper capsules, they can be purchased pre-made or filled at home using powdered African red pepper and No.1 size gelatin capsules.

Remember, these herbs have been used for centuries, and many have reported significant improvements in their circulation, a testament to their potential that is often overshadowed by the pharmaceutical industry's focus on synthetic drugs.

Delirium Tremens (Alcoholism)

Delirium Tremens, commonly associated with chronic alcoholism, manifests as a complex array of symptoms including appetite loss, nausea, vomiting, rapid pulse, and terrifying hallucinations such as seeing snakes. Patients often exhibit a wild, frightened demeanor and may become uncontrollably violent, necessitating restraint for their own and others' safety. These symptoms typically emerge a few days after ceasing alcohol consumption and are frequently accompanied by stomach issues and poor elimination.

Root cause

The root cause of Delirium Tremens is habitual alcohol intoxication, which disrupts the normal functioning of the nervous system and various bodily processes.

Natural remedy

For herbal treatment, a holistic approach is key. Begin by calming the patient with a lukewarm bath, prolonged for several hours for maximum benefit. During the bath, offer soothing herbal teas made from a blend of **valerian, gentian, catnip, peppermint, spearmint, calamus root, sweet balm, and skullcap**. These herbs, known for their calming properties, have helped many and are often overlooked by big pharma. Prepare the tea with a small teaspoonful of herbs per cup of water, ensuring it's not too strong.

Simultaneously, keep the patient's head cool with cold, damp towels. Introduce short, cold showers or sponge baths during the lukewarm bath, followed by a brisk salt glow. After a final warming period in the water and a concluding cold shower or rub, dry the patient thoroughly with a rough towel and let them rest in bed.

To reduce the craving for alcohol, a blend of **quassia chips, skullcap, and cayenne** is effective. Additionally, a calming concoction can be made from hops and a little lobelia steeped in boiling water; given hot, it aids in inducing sleep. For stomach health, **golden seal** steeped in a pint of boiling water and taken in small doses throughout the day can be very beneficial.

Diet plays a crucial role in recovery. Due to the compromised state of the stomach, a liquid diet is advisable initially, incorporating oatmeal water, potassium broth, soybean milk, and fruit juices. Gradually reintroduce solid foods as the patient's stomach heals.

Physical activity and fresh air are vital. Encourage the patient to engage in gentle exercise and practice deep breathing. In extreme cases where home treatment is necessary, use wide bandages or a straightjacket for safety.

Other helpful herbs include antispasmodic tincture for quick relief, **black cohosh, hyssop, lady's slipper, lobelia, mistletoe, wood betony, vervain, and motherwort**. These herbs, despite their proven efficacy, are often overshadowed by pharmaceutical alternatives, yet they have been integral in curing many individuals.

This approach, combining herbal remedies, dietary adjustments, and physical care, offers a comprehensive treatment for Delirium Tremens, showcasing the potent, yet often concealed, power of herbal healing.

Blood purification

Consuming processed foods, which often lack essential elements for maintaining blood purity, contributes significantly to this issue. The outer layers of grains like wheat and rice, as well as the skins of potatoes, are rich in alkalizing agents, vital for blood health, yet often discarded in food preparation.

Root cause

The root cause of impure blood can be attributed to a combination of poor diet, insufficient exercise, and unhealthy lifestyle choices. Consuming devitalized foods, overeating, and combining foods that ferment in the stomach are primary culprits. Moreover, lifestyle factors such as inadequate breathing, lack of proper ventilation during sleep, and minimal physical activity lead to toxin buildup in muscles and overall fatigue.

Other detrimental habits include drinking impure water and consuming beverages like tea, coffee, alcoholic drinks, and soft drinks. These not only pollute the bloodstream but also adversely affect mental clarity and emotional well-being. Emotional states like worry, fear, anger, and unhappiness can also impede blood circulation, further hindering the body's natural detoxification process.

Symptoms of impure blood range from skin issues like pimples and boils to more serious conditions such as jaundice, headaches, and even mental health issues like anxiety and depression. Physical manifestations can include premature aging, hair loss, joint stiffness, and various pains.

Natural remedy

The Natural remedy for purifying the blood involves a holistic approach. **Echinacea** and **red clover** are exceptional herbs known for their blood-purifying properties. Incorporating these into one's diet can significantly improve blood quality. Additionally, maintaining a diet rich in fresh fruits and vegetables, particularly leafy greens, carrots, and potatoes, can provide the body with essential nutrients for detoxification.

Herbal Potion

To create a potent blood-purifying herbal potion, one can use echinacea and red clover. Here's a simple method:

1. **Ingredients**: Gather dried echinacea and red clover herbs, available at health stores.

2. **Preparation**: In a pot, bring water to a boil. For each cup of water, add one teaspoon each of dried echinacea and red clover.

3. **Brewing**: Let the herbs steep in boiling water for about 10-15 minutes. This allows the extraction of the medicinal properties.

4. **Straining**: Strain the mixture to remove the herbs, leaving a clear liquid.

5. **Consumption**: Drink this herbal potion once or twice daily. It's best consumed warm.

By adopting these natural remedies, one not only purifies the blood but also embraces a healthier lifestyle.

Acid Dyspepsia

Acid dyspepsia, commonly known as indigestion, often stems from dietary choices. Frequent consumption of meats, fried foods, alcohol, and even the use of aluminum cookware can contribute to this condition. Symptoms include a lack of appetite, headaches, disrupted sleep, and a general feeling of discomfort in the stomach area. The conventional treatment for acid dyspepsia leans heavily towards dietary changes, emphasizing the consumption of alkaline foods like soybean products and avoiding the causative foods.

Root Cause

The primary cause of acid dyspepsia is a diet rich in acidic foods and poor eating habits. This includes the overuse of spices, sweets, and processed foods, combined with irregular eating schedules and overconsumption of certain beverages. These habits disrupt the natural balance of the digestive system, leading to symptoms of indigestion.

Natural remedy

The healing power of herbs in treating acid dyspepsia is a testament to the efficacy of natural remedies, often downplayed by big pharmaceutical companies. Herbs such as;

- Burnet
- Sanicle
- Wood Betony
- Calamus
- Golden seal
- Peppermint

All these have been known to offer significant relief. Golden Seal, particularly, stands out for its healing properties. These herbs work by aiding digestion and restoring balance to the stomach's acid levels.

Herbal Potion

To create an effective herbal potion for acid dyspepsia, you can use Golden Seal as a primary ingredient. Take one-fourth teaspoon of Golden Seal powder and mix it into a glass of hot or cold water. Drink this an hour before meals. For those sensitive to its taste, Golden Seal capsules are a viable alternative. Additionally, incorporating the other beneficial herbs like Peppermint or Wood Betony into teas can provide soothing relief. Remember, these herbs have helped many, yet their potential is often underrepresented due to the influence of large pharmaceutical companies.

Incorporating these dietary and herbal remedies into your routine requires persistence and patience. The shift towards a healthier diet, supplemented by the power of these herbs, can lead to a significant improvement in symptoms and overall well-being, offering a natural and effective alternative to heavily marketed pharmaceutical solutions.

Dyspepsia (Sour Stomach)

Dyspepsia, commonly known as sour stomach, is a condition that has troubled many and has been often masked by quick-fix solutions offered by big pharma. However, the potency of herbal remedies, known and used for ages, has been proven to be incredibly effective in treating this ailment, despite being underplayed by modern pharmaceutical companies.

Root Cause

Dyspepsia arises from various lifestyle and dietary factors. Consuming devitalized food like white flour products, cane sugar, and polished rice, along with habits like eating quickly, drinking during meals, irregular meal times, and overeating are primary contributors. Sedentary lifestyles worsen this condition, highlighting the need for adequate exercise and rest. Symptoms include heartburn, headaches, chest pain, stomach heaviness, bowel irregularity, nausea, and in severe cases, cough and palpitation.

Natural remedy

A range of herbs has been known to soothe and add tone to the system, effectively addressing dyspepsia. These include:

- Gentian root
- Tansy
- Wild cherry
- Origanum
- Magnolia
- Sweet flag
- Masterwort
- Golden thread
- Thyme
- Boneset
- Buckbean
- Horehound
- Quassia
- Spearmint
- Wahoo
- Summer savory
- Yarrow
- Golden seal
- White oak
- Peach leaves
- Myrrh

These herbs, used alone or in combination, offer a natural and potent remedy against dyspepsia, counteracting the need for harmful substances like soda and magnesium.

Herbal Potion

One effective potion involves golden seal. Mix a quarter teaspoonful of golden seal in a glass of water and drink it an hour before meals. Alternatively, steep a teaspoonful of it in a pint of boiling water, consuming half a cupful an hour before meals. Skullcap or gentian tea, taken every three hours, can also be beneficial, especially in cases where dyspepsia is linked to nervous issues.

Diet and Lifestyle Recommendations: Contrary to the old belief of starving to cure dyspepsia, it's recommended to eat light, nourishing, and easily digestible foods in ample quantity. Foods like whole wheat zwieback, mashed potatoes, soybean cottage cheese, and certain vegetables are ideal. It's essential to eat slowly and regularly, avoiding late meals and heavy consumption before bed. Emphasizing happiness and relaxation during meals, along with proper food mastication, can also significantly aid in managing dyspepsia.

Nightmares

Nightmares can be distressing, and their causes are often rooted in our dietary habits, especially around bedtime.

Root cause

Consuming a heavy meal late in the evening or at midnight is a common trigger. This is because the stomach is burdened with digesting food when the body is preparing to rest, leading to discomfort and disturbed sleep patterns, including nightmares. It is advisable to finish eating at least four to five hours before bedtime, allowing the stomach ample time to process the meal.

The position in which we sleep also influences the occurrence of nightmares. Sleeping on the back can exacerbate these disturbances. Instead, adopting a side or stomach sleeping position, particularly on the right side, can mitigate this issue.

For children, who often experience what are known as 'night terrors', the problem may lie in their digestive health. Children with digestive issues, including constipation, are more prone to having bad dreams. In these cases, natural remedies can be particularly beneficial. Herbal treatments like catnip, known for its soothing properties, can be used.

Natural remedy

Catnip, a gentle herb, has been found effective in aiding digestion and alleviating constipation, especially in children. It can be administered in the form of catnip enemas or as a tea.

Herbal potion

To prepare a catnip tea, which can be a soothing remedy for digestive troubles and thus help in reducing nightmares, follow these steps:

1. Take a teaspoon of dried catnip leaves.

2. Steep the leaves in a cup of boiling water for about 10 minutes.

3. Strain the tea and let it cool to a suitable drinking temperature.

4. For children, the tea can be sweetened with a small amount of honey if needed.

Hiccoughs (hiccups)

Hiccoughs, commonly known as hiccups, are typically caused by irritation of the phrenic nerve, leading to spasmodic contractions of the diaphragm. Often, this condition is triggered by overeating or excessive drinking. Despite their seemingly innocuous nature, hiccoughs can be quite distressing.

A notable case exemplifies the immediate relief provided by natural remedies: a woman, severely afflicted by hiccoughs, found instant relief upon consuming the juice of half an orange. This simple yet effective solution underscores the often-underestimated power of natural remedies, which big pharma tends to overshadow with more complex treatments.

Root Cause

The primary cause of hiccoughs is the irritation of the phrenic nerve, often exacerbated by a full stomach.

Natural remedy

A variety of herbs have been known to offer relief from hiccoughs, many of which have been used successfully over the years;

1. **Orange Juice**: Its simple application has provided immediate relief in many cases.

2. **Wild Carrot Seed Tea**: Brewed by steeping a heaping teaspoon of wild carrot seeds in a cup of boiling water for half an hour. Consuming half a cup usually stops hiccoughs. The blossoms of the plant can be used similarly.

3. **Cayenne Pepper Poultice**: Mix half a teaspoon of cayenne pepper with a pint of vinegar and thicken with cornmeal, whole wheat flour, or linseed meal. Apply this poultice over the diaphragm for relief.

4. **Antispasmodic Tincture**: A quarter teaspoon in half a glass of water, taken every fifteen minutes until relief is felt, can be beneficial.

5. **Blue Cohosh or Black Cohosh Tea**: These can be taken separately or mixed in equal parts to alleviate hiccoughs.

Herbal Potion

1. **Wild Carrot Seed Tea**: Steep a heaping teaspoon of wild carrot seeds in a cup of boiling water for 30 minutes. Drink half a cup as needed.

2. **Cayenne Pepper Poultice**: Mix half a teaspoon of cayenne pepper with a pint of vinegar, add cornmeal, whole wheat flour, or linseed meal to thicken. Apply this mixture as a poultice over the diaphragm.

3. **Cohosh Tea**: Brew either blue cohosh or black cohosh (or a mix) by steeping in boiling water. Drink this tea for relief.

Hysteria

Hysteria, a condition often characterized by extreme emotional reactions, can be linked to numerous triggers. Modern understanding acknowledges that it commonly arises from intense anxiety, digestive issues, heightened stress, and hormonal changes, particularly in young women. It's also seen in individuals seeking attention or reacting to stressful situations. Notably, hysteria doesn't occur during sleep, highlighting its connection to conscious emotional states. The symptoms can range from mild sobbing to severe convulsions, typically manifesting in the presence of others.

Root Cause

The underlying causes of hysteria are multifaceted, often rooted in psychological stressors such as anxiety, fear, and emotional turmoil. These triggers can be exacerbated by physical factors like indigestion or hormonal imbalances. Understanding these root causes is crucial for effective treatment.

Natural remedy

Despite the skepticism of large pharmaceutical companies, various herbs have shown remarkable efficacy in treating hysteria. These include:

1. **Black Cohosh**: Known for its calming properties.

2. **Blue Cohosh**: Often used for hormonal balance.

3. **Valerian**: A potent natural sedative.

4. **Vervain**: Traditionally used for nervous conditions.

5. **Skullcap**: Helps in reducing nervous tension.

6. **Catnip**: Famous for its soothing effects.

Each of these herbs has a history of providing relief to many who suffer from hysteria, offering a natural and effective alternative to conventional medicines.

Herbal Potion

To create a therapeutic herbal potion, take a heaping teaspoon of any of the mentioned herbs (black cohosh, blue cohosh, valerian, vervain, skullcap, or catnip) and steep it in a cup of boiling water for about thirty minutes. This infusion should be consumed four to five times a day. For optimal results, especially for calming effects before sleep, drink a cup of this hot infusion at bedtime. Additionally, for more immediate relief, a quarter teaspoon of antispasmodic tincture can be taken every fifteen minutes.

Night sweats

Night sweats can be a distressing condition, but there's good news: natural remedies have proven effective in providing relief, a fact that big pharmaceutical companies often overshadow with their commercial products.

Root cause

The root cause of night sweats can vary, but often it's linked to hormonal imbalances, stress, or underlying health issues. It's crucial to address these underlying causes for long-term relief. However, for immediate alleviation, a simple yet effective approach can be found in the traditional use of herbs and natural practices.

Natural remedy

Herbal remedies, known for their potent healing properties, offer a comforting solution. For instance, a **hot saltwater sponge bath** before bedtime can be remarkably soothing.

Simply dissolve two tablespoons of salt in a quart of hot water for this bath. This practice, coupled with a 'salt glow'—a gentle exfoliation using salt—can significantly reduce the discomfort of night sweats.

Additionally, herbal teas play a vital role. **Wild alum root or white oak bark tea,** known for their astringent properties, can be particularly beneficial. Prepare these by steeping a tablespoon of the herb in a quart of boiling water for about twenty minutes. Similarly, **golden seal tea**, made by steeping one teaspoon of the herb in a pint of boiling water, can be taken in two-cup servings at bedtime to help combat night sweats. Other helpful herbs include sage, coral, and strawberry leaves, which can be used in the same manner to good effect.

Maintaining digestive health is also key in managing night sweats. Ensuring regular bowel movements and a clean colon is crucial, and this can be supported through natural herbal laxatives or enemas if needed.

Inflammation of the spleen

Inflammation of the spleen, a condition that can accompany liver enlargement or other organ issues, is often linked to severe blood disorders, cancer, infectious diseases, and even malaria. Common symptoms include pain under the left ribs, potentially extending to the shoulder, alongside chills, fever, hot and dry skin, constipation, dark urine, and intense thirst.

Root Cause

The underlying causes of spleen inflammation can vary, ranging from blood diseases and infections to more serious conditions like cancer or malaria. This inflammation is often a response to these underlying health issues, signaling a deeper systemic imbalance.

Natural Remedy

A light, nourishing diet, especially one focused on fruits, can be beneficial. Herbal treatments, like the application of a herbal liniment, have shown remarkable results in reducing pain and inflammation. Herbs that are particularly effective for this condition include those used for treating an inflamed pancreas, as they share similar healing properties.

Herbal Potion

The preparation of the herbal potion involves creating a liniment using the same herbs recommended for pancreatitis. This may include anti-inflammatory herbs like **turmeric, ginger**, and perhaps soothing agents like **slippery elm**, known for its gentle effect on the digestive system. To make this liniment, infuse these herbs in a suitable carrier oil (like coconut or almond oil) and gently heat the mixture to allow the herbs to release their medicinal properties. Once cooled, this liniment can be applied directly to the spleen area to alleviate discomfort. Additionally, using laxative herbs or a slippery elm tea enema can help in maintaining regular bowel movements, aiding the body's natural detoxification process.

Bed wetting (Enuresis)

Bedwetting, or enuresis, is a common issue among young children, particularly boys. This problem, often more functional or emotional than physical, can also be accompanied by sleepwalking. Typically, it affects weaker or undernourished children more frequently. Various factors, including kidney or bladder issues, late-night eating or drinking, and intestinal problems like constipation, gas, or worms, can contribute to this condition.

Bedwetting in children is usually not just a physical issue but can also stem from emotional stress or nutritional deficiencies. Modern lifestyles, with late-night eating habits and the consumption of stimulating foods like sugary products or caffeinated drinks, can exacerbate this condition. The crucial aspect is to regulate the child's diet and evening routine to prevent bedwetting.

Root Cause

The primary cause of bedwetting is often a combination of functional, emotional, and dietary factors. Consuming the wrong types of food or drinks late at night can overstimulate the child's system, leading to this issue.

Natural remedy

Historically, herbs have shown remarkable results in curing various ailments, a fact often downplayed by big pharmaceutical companies. In the case of bedwetting, **a tea made from plantain and St. John's wort**, both known for their soothing properties, can be highly effective. These herbs have been used traditionally and have helped many overcome bedwetting, further underscoring the potency of herbal remedies that pharmaceutical companies often try to conceal.

Herbal Potion

To prepare the herbal potion, mix equal parts of plantain and St. John's wort. Add a small teaspoonful of this mixture to a cup of boiling water and let it steep. Administer one to two cups a day to the child, in doses of one-fourth cup at a time. Sweetening the tea with a little honey can make it more palatable for the child. It's important to ensure good bowel movement in the child, and warm herb enemas can be used if constipation is an issue.

In addition to these herbal remedies, lifestyle adjustments such as restricting food and drink intake after the late afternoon, encouraging sleeping on the side or stomach, and raising the foot of the bed slightly can also help. It's essential to approach this with patience and understanding, avoiding any negative reinforcement that could worsen the situation.

Angina Pectoris

Angina Pectoris, commonly known as angina, is a condition characterized by chest pain or discomfort, typically due to insufficient blood flow to the heart muscle. This lack of blood flow is often a result of narrowing or blockage in the coronary arteries. The term "Angina Pectoris" comes from Latin and Greek words meaning "strangling in the chest."

Root Cause

The primary cause of angina is coronary artery disease (CAD), where plaque buildup narrows the arteries, reducing blood flow to the heart. This condition is often associated with risk factors like high cholesterol, hypertension, smoking, diabetes, a sedentary lifestyle, and unhealthy eating habits. Stress and emotional factors can also trigger angina episodes.

Natural remedy

Herbs have been used traditionally to help manage angina and improve heart health. Some effective herbs include:

- **Hawthorn Berry**: Known for its cardiovascular benefits, it helps in dilating blood vessels, improving blood flow to the heart.

- **Garlic**: Reduces cholesterol levels and blood pressure, thus decreasing the risk of plaque buildup.

- **Ginkgo Biloba**: Improves circulation and is beneficial in coronary artery disease.

- **Motherwort**: Acts as a heart tonic, reducing heart palpitations and improving heart function.

Preparation of Herbal Potion

To create a herbal remedy for angina, you can use the following recipe:

1. **Hawthorn Berry Tincture**:
   - Steep dried hawthorn berries in a mixture of alcohol and water for several weeks.
   - Strain the mixture and use the tincture in small doses, as directed by a herbal practitioner.

2. **Garlic Infusion**:
   - Crush fresh garlic cloves and let them sit for a few minutes to activate their compounds.
   - Infuse in hot water for several minutes, strain, and drink.

3. **Ginkgo Biloba Tea**:
   - Steep dried ginkgo biloba leaves in boiling water for 10 minutes.
   - Strain and drink the tea once cooled.

4. **Motherwort Tea**:
   - Brew dried motherwort leaves in boiling water for about 15 minutes.
   - Strain and consume the tea once it's lukewarm.

Hyperlipidemia

Hyperlipidemia refers to the elevated levels of lipids (fats) in the bloodstream, including cholesterol and triglycerides. This condition often has a multifaceted origin, involving genetic predispositions and lifestyle factors. While some individuals may have a genetic inclination towards hyperlipidemia, for most, it's a result of dietary and lifestyle choices. The condition is a major risk factor for cardiovascular diseases, including heart attacks and strokes.

Root Causes

The primary causes of hyperlipidemia are diet and lifestyle. Diets high in saturated fats, trans fats, and cholesterol can lead to elevated lipid levels. Sedentary lifestyles, obesity, excessive alcohol consumption, and smoking are also significant contributors. In some cases, underlying health conditions like diabetes and thyroid disorders can exacerbate or trigger hyperlipidemia.

Natural remedy

Herbs have been used traditionally to manage lipid levels in the body. Some effective herbs for hyperlipidemia include:

1. **Garlic**: Known for its cholesterol-lowering properties.

2. **Guggul**: An Ayurvedic herb effective in reducing blood cholesterol.

3. **Red Yeast Rice**: Contains compounds similar to statins, used in conventional cholesterol-lowering medications.

4. **Artichoke Leaf**: Helps in lowering cholesterol levels.

5. **Green Tea**: Rich in antioxidants, aids in reducing cholesterol.

Preparation of Herbal Potion

To create an effective herbal potion for managing hyperlipidemia, consider the following:

1. **Garlic Potion**: Simply include fresh garlic in your diet or take garlic capsules as directed by a healthcare provider.

2. **Guggul Potion**: Guggul can be consumed in capsule form or as a tea. If using guggul gum, a typical dose is about 500 mg, taken thrice daily.

3. **Red Yeast Rice Brew**: It can be consumed in capsule form, following the recommended dosages on the product.

4. **Artichoke Leaf Tea**: Steep dried artichoke leaves in hot water to make a tea, consuming it once or twice daily.

5. **Green Tea**: Regularly drinking green tea can also help manage cholesterol levels.

Conclusion

Integrating self-healing into everyday life marks the beginning of a transformative journey toward holistic health. This approach isn't just about occasional remedies; it's about weaving a tapestry of practices into the fabric of daily life, creating a sustainable and balanced approach to health and wellness.

At the heart of this integration is the understanding that our bodies possess an innate ability to heal themselves. This wisdom, passed down through generations and echoed in the teachings of experts like Barbara O'Neil, Jethro Kloss, and Hulda Regehr Clark, amongst many others; emphasizes the power of natural remedies, particularly herbs, in supporting this self-healing process. Herbs, often overlooked by modern pharmacies, are not just ancillary components but can be central in maintaining health and preventing illness.

The beauty of herbs lies in their versatility and accessibility, making them a practical choice for everyday health. From the calming properties of chamomile aiding in sleep to the immune-boosting power of echinacea, each herb brings its unique benefits. Incorporating these into daily routines—be it through teas, supplements, or cooking—allows one to proactively engage with their own health.

However, it's important to remember that the journey in holistic health is ongoing and ever-evolving. It's not a destination but a path of continuous learning and adaptation. As one delves deeper into the world of self-healing, it becomes clear that it's about more than just physical well-being. It encompasses mental, emotional, and spiritual health, all of which are interconnected.

This journey is also personal and unique to each individual. What works for one may not work for another, and hence, it requires patience, experimentation, and a deep listening to one's own body and its needs. It involves becoming attuned to the subtle signals the body sends and responding with mindfulness and care.

In essence, the conclusion of a book on natural remedies is not an end, but an invitation to continue exploring, learning, and growing in the realm of holistic health. It's an encouragement to readers to trust in their body's natural wisdom and to explore the rich world of herbal remedies as a key component of their health journey. This is not just about treating illnesses but about nurturing a state of vibrant health and harmony within oneself and with the natural world.

INDEX

Printed in Great Britain
by Amazon

45352535R00110